The COSTS of WORKER DISLOCATION

Louis Jacobson
Robert LaLonde
Daniel Sullivan

1993

W. E. UPJOHN INSTITUTE for Employment Research
Kalamazoo, Michigan

Library of Congress Cataloging-in-Publication Data

Jacobson, Louis S.
  The costs of workers dislocation / Louis S. Jacobson, Robert J. LaLonde,
Daniel G. Sullivan.
      p.   cm.
  Includes bibliographical references and index.
  ISBN 0-88099-144-5, — ISBN 0-88099-143-7 (pbk.)
  1. Displaced workers—Pennsylvania—Economic conditions.
  I. LaLonde, Robert   II. Sullivan, Daniel..
  III. Title.
  HD5708.55.U62P44   1993
  331.13'73'09748—dc20   93-23613
                                                             CIP

The facts presented in this study and the observations and viewpoints expressed are the sole responsibility of the author. They do not necessarily represent positions of the W.E. Upjohn Institute for Employment Research.

Cover design by J.R. Underhill.
Index prepared by Shirley Kessel.
Printed in the United States of America.

Acknowledgments

We thank the Pennsylvania Department of Labor and Industry for providing the data used in this monograph and for technical assistance. We also appreciate the research support provided by the Allegheny County Department of Planning, the Graduate School of Business at the University of Chicago, the W. E. Upjohn Institute for Employment Research, and the Industrial Relations Section at Princeton University. The views expressed herein are not necessarily those of the Federal Reserve Bank of Chicago or the Federal Reserve System.

We have benefited from helpful comments by Joseph Altonji, David Card, Matthew Cunningham, Robert Gibbons, John Ham, Daniel Hamermesh, James Heckman, Bruce Meyer, Canice Prendergast, Christopher Ruhm, Jeffrey Smith, Robert Topel, and seminar participants at the University of Chicago, the W. E. Upjohn Institute for Employment Research, Princeton University, the University of Illinois, the Federal Reserve Bank of Chicago, the National Bureau of Economic Research, the Board of Governors of the Federal Reserve System, the University of Pittsburgh, the University of Iowa, Texas A & M University, and Johns Hopkins University. We also thank Melissa Barnhart and Carolyn Thies for excellent research assistance.

Finally and most importantly, we thank our families for their patience and support while this monograph was being prepared.

Authors

Louis S. Jacobson, a senior economist at Westat Incorporated, was formerly a senior economist at the W. E. Upjohn Institute. He received his Ph.D. from Northwestern University. Dr. Jacobson's research has focused on the nature and consequences of changes in the structure of employment and the effectiveness of compensation mechanisms such as the Trade Adjustment Assistance program. He has also studied the effectiveness of the Employment Service as an aid to displaced workers.

Robert J. LaLonde is associate professor of industrial relations at the Graduate School of Business of the University of Chicago. He served previously as a senior staff economist for the Council of Economic Advisers. Dr. LaLonde received his Ph.D. from Princeton University. His previous research has been on the evaluation of training programs, the employment effects of unions and reasons for decline in unionization rates, and immigration (rates of assimilation and effects on native workers).

Daniel G. Sullivan, a senior research economist and research officer with the Federal Reserve Bank of Chicago, received his Ph.D. in economics from Princeton University. He is also a visiting scholar with the Center for Urban Affairs and Policy Research at Northwestern University. In addition to his research on displaced workers, he has published articles on the effect of subsidized training programs on participant employment rates, the labor market for professional nurses, and the cigarette industry.

Contents

List of Tables

List of Figures

The
COSTS
of
WORKER
DISLOCATION

1
Introduction

The high U.S. unemployment rates brought on by the recent recession have refocused the attention of policymakers on the plight of displaced workers—workers whose job losses result from layoffs and plant closings associated with economic restructuring. The causes of such restructuring are varied and include shifts in product demand, changes in technology, or even poor management. Although the economy as a whole benefits when restructuring occurs, most would agree that some costs are imposed on the workers who lose their jobs. There is, however, a substantial range of opinion about the magnitude of those costs. Some view displacement as a temporary setback from which workers easily recover, while others believe it to be nearly catastrophic, causing large, permanent reductions in workers' earnings. In this monograph we add to the existing literature by more precisely estimating the magnitude and temporal pattern of the earnings losses of displaced workers.[1]

In addition to economic restructuring, changes in public policy may also lead to worker dislocation. Concern over that possibility has been prominent in the debate over the free-trade agreement with Canada and Mexico.[2] It is clear that consumers will benefit from such an agreement. But, some workers are likely to lose their jobs as a result of increased competition. Likewise, controversies over environmental protection often involve similar trade-offs. The benefits associated with protecting the spotted owls in Pacific Northwest forests,[3] the salmon in Washington State rivers,[4] and the snaildarter in Tennessee waterways[5] all come at the cost of lost jobs. As with economic restructuring, society as a whole may benefit from such public policies, but costs are imposed on the workers who lose their jobs.

There are two reasons why policymakers are interested in the magnitude of losses suffered by workers. First, whether they actually will want to intervene in the economy may depend on the magnitude of losses borne by displaced workers. Such considerations are especially likely to arise when policymakers undertake interventions to protect the environment. In such instances, it is often not clear whether the benefits of their actions exceed the costs. A second reason for such interest in the losses of displaced workers is that even when, as in most cases of proposed trade liberalization, society derives net benefits from the intervention, policymakers may want to compensate those who are displaced. They may want to provide this compensation because they believe that "fairness" requires it or because they believe that compensating displaced workers is the only politically feasible way to bring about change.[6]

1.1 Policies to Aid Displaced Workers

Policymakers have, in fact, long recognized that dislocation may be costly and have attempted to ameliorate the losses of displaced workers through a series of federally funded programs that have provided these workers with both cash and retraining services. In the late 1950s and early 1960s, the concern was primarily with workers whose joblessness resulted from automation.[7] The Area Redevelopment Act of 1959 provided training and relocation assistance to such workers. That legislation was followed by the Manpower Development and Training Act of 1962 which provided expanded classroom and on-the-job training opportunities to displaced workers. In the 1970s, concern shifted from the effects of automation to those of foreign competition. As a result, in 1974 Congress relaxed eligibility requirements for Trade Adjustment Assistance under the Trade Act (Leigh 1990, pp. 92-94). Those changes allowed the Secretary of Labor to authorize compensation for large numbers of workers who had lost their jobs as a result of import competition rather than explicit trade liberalizations.

More recently, policymakers' attention has been drawn to what are perceived to be the special problems experienced by workers displaced from the manufacturing sector—a sector that experienced a permanent employment loss of approximately 1.5 million net jobs during the 1980s (Economic Report of the President 1991: 334, table B-43). The high unemployment rates experienced by such job losses are largely due to substantially longer unemployment spells (Murphy and Topel 1987, pp. 24-26). Evidence indicating that prime-age males were having difficulty adjusting to their job losses was an important consideration in Congress' decision to include a job training component in the TAA program and to expand services under the Job Training Partnership Act of 1982 with the Economic Dislocation and Worker Adjustment Assistance Act of 1988 (Leigh 1990: 93-94). As a result of that legislation, during fiscal year 1991, the federal government spent nearly $1 billion specifically to aid displaced workers (U.S. Office of Management and Budget 1991).

As we discuss more fully in subsequent chapters, the most effective mix of cash subsidies, retraining opportunities, and job search assistance depends critically on such factors as the relative importance of unemployment in determining displaced worker losses and whether the displaced are likely to find work similar to their former jobs. The research presented in this monograph is intended to shed light on these questions and thus to aid in the formulation of cost effective assistance programs. We also investigate whether the special concern for displaced manufacturing workers is warranted by the uniqueness of their experiences.

1.2 Why Job Loss May Be Costly in the Long Run

Clearly, job loss adversely affects workers in the short term if they are forced into unemployment while searching for a new job. However, longer term losses can only result from displacement if workers' earnings with their former employers exceeded what they could have earned with other potential employers. There are several reasons why workers could have received such earnings premiums on their former jobs. First, firm and industry earnings premiums may result when jobs are covered by a collective bargaining agreement. A great deal of evidence indicates that unionization raises workers' wages (Lewis 1986, pp. 9, 125-28). Further, unionized firms may find it profitable to maintain relative wage differentials between various classes of workers and thus may respond to the unionization of one segment of their workforce by paying wage premiums to all their employees (Hirsch and Addison 1986). Similarly, these earnings premiums may become industrywide when the industry's nonunion firms, fearing unionization, respond to collective bargaining settlements of rivals by raising their own workers' pay. Therefore, the earnings loss associated with worker separations depends partially on the magnitude of the union wage gap and on whether displaced workers are able to find new jobs in similarly unionized industries.

Earnings premiums may also arise in competitive (nonunion) labor markets if workers have skills that enhance their productivity with their current employer, but are less valued by other potential employers. For instance, both firms and workers may desire long-term employment relationships in order to recoup investments in skills that are specific to the firms. The most effective mechanism for assuring the continuance of such relationships is for the firm to pay workers more than they would receive elsewhere (Becker 1975). Moreover, paying earnings premiums may be profitable even when workers have not acquired their specialized skills on the job. Some employees' skills may simply be well matched to a particular employer. In this case, the resulting earnings premiums reflect the considerable costs incurred both by the firm when recruiting and evaluating new employees and by workers when seeking appropriate employment (Jovanovic 1979).

A third reason why earnings premiums may exist is that productivity of workers may depend directly on their pay. For instance, earnings premiums may induce employees to work harder and may discourage them from quitting. In this case, it is profitable for firms to offer premiums as long as their costs are offset by increased productivity. However, offering premiums cannot always be profitable. Otherwise, all firms would attempt to pay them and there would be no premiums. Circumstances that make paying premiums attractive include those involving teamwork and those where monitoring workers' performance is difficult. When workers who earn premiums lose their jobs as a result of restructuring, they are likely to either have to take a new job where earnings premia are not paid or wait in a long queue for a job similar to their old one. In either case they will suffer earnings declines.[8]

A final reason why job loss may result in substantial earnings reductions is the prevalence in certain sectors of the labor market of employment practices that preclude lateral entry. That is, in order to induce employees to work hard and make the necessary investments to enhance their productivity, certain kinds of firms may commit themselves to a promotion-from-within policy. Under such a system, new hires always start in entry-level positions, and those who perform well move into higher paying jobs. Should the successful workers be displaced by economic restructuring and subsequently accept employment with a similar firm, they will begin in jobs farther down the promotion ladder. This effective demotion is likely to be associated with earnings losses (Lazear 1981).

Each of the foregoing reasons for why workers may receive earnings premiums implies that workers displaced as a result of economic restructuring or public policy changes may experience earnings losses even after finding new employment. These theories do not, however, provide much guidance about the magnitude of the resulting losses. In addition, they differ in their implications for how long these losses might last. In some cases, such as when the earnings declines result from lost union premiums, they will be permanent. In other cases, such as when the declines result from terminating a good worker-firm match, they may diminish with time. These possibilities indicate that it is important to study how the magnitude of those losses vary with time following workers' separations.

1.3   This Study's Objectives and Findings

In this monograph, we examine the magnitude and temporal pattern of earnings losses suffered by a group of experienced workers who separated from their firms in the early and mid-1980s. We estimate these losses by comparing workers' postdisplacement earnings to their expected earnings had they not been displaced. We also examine how earnings losses depend on various characteristics of the workers and their former employers.

This study is distinguished from others that have examined similar questions by its use of a newly available data set derived from the administrative records of the State of Pennsylvania. This data set contains the quarterly earnings histories of a large number of workers covering the period 1974 through 1986 merged with employment information about their firms. These data have several advantages over those used in previous studies. First, because our sample is larger than others that have been used to examine the losses of displaced workers, we are able to obtain estimates for more narrowly defined groups of workers and thus are better able to determine the characteristics of workers most severely affected by job loss. Second, because the earnings histories stretch over a longer period of time than those used in previous studies, we are able to learn more about the long-term consequences of job loss. The longer panel also allows us to observe the earnings of displaced workers well before their separations and thus greatly improves our ability to forecast what their earnings would have been had they not been displaced. Third, because we have data on workers' firms, we can examine how the costs of displacement depend on their firm's economic health. And finally, because we also have a large sample of workers who were not displaced during the 1980s, we can construct comparison groups that improve our estimates of how the earnings of displaced workers would have grown in the absence of job loss.

There are, of course, also some disadvantages associated with our use of administrative data. First, we do not know for certain whether a particular separation was a layoff, a discharge for cause, or a quit. The latter two classes of worker separations do not reflect the effects of the economic restructuring that we wish to study, and it is unlikely that they have the same consequences for workers' subsequent earnings.[9] As indicated by the literature, however, quits and discharges for cause decline sharply as tenure with the firm increases (Mincer and Jovanovic 1981). Thus, because we limit our analysis to workers with six or more years of tenure, our sample of separations should consist largely of involuntary layoffs. Moreover, with our data it is possible to identify groups of workers leaving firms experiencing large employment declines. Such separations almost certainly are the result of economic restructuring.[10]

A second disadvantage of our use of administrative data is that we possess only limited demographic information on the workers we study. Our sample is selected so that we know workers' gender and year of birth. However, we do not have access to such standard human capital measures as years of education, nor do we know workers' occupations. Because we rely completely on estimation techniques that exploit our data's longitudinal nature, this lack of demographic information does not lead to any bias in our estimates of the average losses suffered by displaced workers. However, lack of data does prevent us from analyzing how earnings losses depend on factors such as education and occupation. Similarly, our lack of a measure of hours worked prevents us from studying how displacement separately affects hours of work and wages.

Like other worker dislocation studies, our findings indicate that experienced workers incur substantial earnings losses immediately after they separate from their firms. Much of this initial loss results from increased unemployment. We also show, however, that these losses are generally shared by workers in all demographic groups and most industrial sectors, and more important, that they persist for several years after displacement. Even in the fifth year following separations, we estimate that annual losses of displaced workers average more than $6,500, an amount equal to more than 25 percent of their predisplacement earnings. During the first six years following their job losses, we estimate that their discounted earnings losses totaled $41,000. That estimate holds for both older and younger workers, varies only modestly for workers displaced from different industries, and is only slightly lower for women.

Moreover, we find that the earnings of displaced workers begin to diverge from their expected levels two to three years before they leave their firms. This divergence appears to result from reduced hours, cuts in real wages, and increased temporary layoffs in the period before permanent separations. Temporary layoffs, in particular, account for a significant fraction of predisplacement earnings declines. We argue below that these losses likely result from firms' responses to economic restructuring or to policy changes, and therefore they should be included as part of the costs of worker dislocation. When we include their preseparation losses as well as a reasonable estimate of their losses more than five years after separation, the present value of their losses rises to approximately $80,000.

One implication of our findings is that existing government programs do not, and probably cannot, compensate for more than a small portion of displaced workers' losses. One reason for this is that most of the losses accumulate after they are reemployed, and unemployment insurance benefits, the main form of assistance for displaced workers, do not cover such losses. A second reason that the effectiveness of existing programs is limited is that earnings losses are large even when displaced workers find new jobs in their old industries. As we argue below, this suggests that existing employment and training programs, including job search assistance, though they might be cost effective, cannot entirely eliminate experienced workers' losses. Another implication of our findings is that, instead of bolstering existing programs, it may be more efficient to assist displaced workers by introducing an income or earnings subsidy.

The remainder of this monograph proceeds as follows: In chapter 2, we review the previous literature on dislocation, with special emphasis on the empirical methods used in these studies and on the evidence of long-term effects of displacement. In chapter 3, we introduce our longitudinal data on Pennsylvania workers and identify several issues associated with estimating earnings losses. In chapter 4, we discuss the statistical methodologies underlying our formal estimates of earnings losses. In chapter 5, we present estimates of the earnings losses incurred by all experienced workers separating from their firms during the early and mid-1980s. In chapter 6, we restrict our focus to workers leaving firms experiencing closings and mass layoffs and show how earnings losses depend on the economic health of workers' former firms, on their former industry, on local labor market conditions, and on whether they found new jobs in their old industrial sectors. Chapter 7 summarizes our findings and discusses their implications for public policy.

NOTES

1. As noted, there is some difference of opinion on this issue. On the one hand, Michael Boskin, Chairman of the President's Council of Economic Advisers under President Bush, has asserted that the overwhelming bulk of people laid off during the most recent recession would eventually find jobs that pay something close to their former wages (*Chicago Tribune*, September 29, 1991, p. 2). On the other hand, reflecting on debates over policies to aid the jobless, Rudy Kuzel, currently President of United Auto Workers Local 72 in Kenosha, Wisconsin, remarked that, "They cut people's throat in this country and then they argue about what size Band-Aid to apply" (*Chicago Tribune*, October 2, 1991, p. 15). We suspect that such fundamental disagreement over the seriousness of job loss underlies much debate over appropriate public policy.

2. See, for example, James Carville, "Help Those Whom NAFTA Will Hurt," *Washington Post*, July 25, 1993, Section C, p. 7; Elaine S. Povich, "Trade Pact Conditions," *Chicago Tribune*, April 30, 1991, Business Section, pp. 1-5; and D. Corn, "Harkin's Bid," *The Nation*, July 29-August 5, 1991, p. 158. A similar debate occurred when the free-trade agreement with Canada was ratified. See *New York Times*, June 27, 1988, Section D, p. 10; and *New York Times*, January 3, 1988, Section A, p. 12.

3. For instance, in the case of the spotted owls, the costs of preserving their habitat is borne disproportionately by workers in the lumber industry. See "Clinton Pledges 'Balanced' Solution to Forest Policy Crisis in 2 Months," *Washington Post,* May 13, 1993, Section 1, p. 2; and "U.S.: Saving Rare Owl Would Cost 40,000 Jobs," *Chicago Tribune,* April 30, 1991, Section 1, p. 14.

4. See *New York Times,* April 1, 1991, Section A, p. 1; and *Wall Street Journal,* May 16, 1991, Section A, p. 16.

5. See *Science,* February 23, 1979, p. 730; and *Time,* October 8, 1979, p. 105.

6. See Owen and Braeutigam (1978) for a discussion of the possibility that without some mechanism for compensating those who are hurt by regulatory change, all such change would be blocked; and see Cordes and Weisbrod (1979) for evidence that increasing levels of compensation to those who are adversely affected can increase the rate at which public highway building projects are undertaken.

7. See President's Advisory Committee on Labor Management Policy (1962).

8. For alternative versions of this basic model, see Stiglitz (1974); Akerlof (1982); and Shapiro and Stiglitz (1984).

9. See McLaughlin (1991).

10. Indeed, our data probably allow us to identify displaced workers *more* accurately than data sets such as the Bureau of Labor Statistics Displaced Workers Survey, which relies on worker self-reports and is, therefore, subject to recall biases and perhaps to misreporting due to the stigma associated with being discharged for cause. See Topel (1990).

2
Evidence from Earlier Studies of the Costs of Worker Dislocation

Our study of the costs of worker dislocation builds on a substantial body of earlier research. The primary aim of this chapter is to describe the methodology and findings from earlier worker dislocation studies. While many of those studies focused primarily on issues beyond the scope of this monograph, they often directly or indirectly examined the earnings costs of dislocated worker job losses and the factors that made those losses costly. Our survey is not comprehensive, but instead reflects our interest in (1) the long-run effect of worker dislocation on earnings, and (2) the different strategies used to estimate the costs of worker dislocation, especially how those estimates depend on the choice of a comparison group and on the availability of a long predisplacement earnings history. We do not summarize every study of worker displacement; instead, we limit our survey to research that characterizes the methodology and findings from a broader set of studies.

The chapter is divided into six sections. In section 2.1, we briefly comment on findings from the many case studies of the effects of plant closings on displaced workers. In section 2.2, we survey the findings and methodologies used in a series of studies sponsored by the U.S. Department of Labor's Bureau of International Labor Affairs (ILAB). The purpose, data, and methodology of the studies were often similar to our own. Accordingly, our review of them is relatively extensive. In section 2.3, we summarize the evidence on earnings losses of displaced workers derived from the Displaced Workers Survey (DWS). In section 2.4, we assess recent studies that examine the relationship between earnings losses and predisplacement tenure of workers. In section 2.5, we examine the merits of using cross-sectional versus longitudinal data when estimating the costs of worker dislocation. Finally, some concluding remarks follow in section 2.6.

2.1 Lessons From Case Studies

Surveys such as that by Gordus, Jarley, and Ferman (1981) provide a comprehensive examination of case studies of how plant closings affect the subsequent earnings of workers. These studies usually examine the losses experienced by unionized workers when their plants shut down in already depressed areas. Among the best-known studies are those of dislocated workers in the meat packing and auto industries, but other studies examine the effects of dislocation on primarily female workforces from the textile and electronic assembly industries and on workers from firms in defense-related industries. Most often these case studies have found that displaced workers incurred long periods of joblessness following their displacements. They also have found that earnings losses were greatest for older, unionized, high-wage, blue-collar men, and for those residing in areas where their entire industry was in decline or areas with relatively isolated labor markets.

For our purposes, these case studies suffer from several shortcomings. Among their principal deficiencies is that they typically characterize "worst-case" scenarios. The plants studied were chosen because it was believed that the earnings losses would be large. Therefore, the workers studied may not be representative of the population of dislocated workers, many of whom left firms or plants that remained open. Another shortcoming of these studies is that they were based on interviews only a year or two after worker separations. As a result, little was learned about long-term earnings losses of workers following their displacements.

2.2 Studies of Trade-Impacted Workers

Concern about the costs of job loss stemming from heightened foreign competition prompted ILAB to sponsor a series of studies that dealt in part with the costs of worker dislocation. Several of those studies focused on workers who received Trade Adjustment Assistance (TAA).[1] Other studies examined the costs of declining demand on workers in trade-sensitive manufacturing industries who did not necessarily receive TAA.

The characteristics of workers in the ILAB studies often differed from those in subsequent studies using the Displaced Workers Survey because ILAB was concerned about both permanent job loss and temporary job loss followed by recall to the same employer. Under the Trade Expansion Act of 1962, TAA recipients had to demonstrate that their layoffs resulted from the lifting of import restrictions, but they did not need to show that their job loss was permanent. The Trade Act of 1974 relaxed those eligibility requirements so that unemployed workers had only to show that imports contributed to their layoffs. In addition, the Act increased both the maximum potential duration of unemployment insurance (UI) payments and the levels of those payments.

Prior to the 1974 legislative changes, few workers received TAA. Those who did were predominantly from plants that closed in the relatively low-wage footwear, textiles, and electronic assembly industries. Accordingly, in comparing the characteristics of TAA recipients to other job losers, Neumann (1978b) noted that "(a) broad generalization would be that trade-impacted workers were older, less educated, semiskilled or unskilled, and had a lot of years on the job. It is precisely such workers who could be expected to have a difficult time finding another job." By contrast, workers who received TAA under the 1974 Act included younger unemployed workers from the high-wage steel and auto industries, 85 percent of whom were ultimately recalled.[2]

Neumann (1978b) found evidence of substantial earnings losses as measured by the difference between displaced TAA recipients' post- and predisplacement earnings. In particular, he found from a survey of pre-1974 TAA recipients that both males and females experienced losses approaching 25 percent of their former earnings. For purposes of assessing the long-term effects of displacement, this study's primary shortcomings were that it did not use a comparison group of nondisplaced workers and it did not control for the time between the date of a worker's job loss and the interview date. As a result, it was impossible to infer how actual postdisplacement earnings compared to what they would have been in the absence of displacement and whether the substantial earnings reductions observed were permanent or temporary.

Corson and Nicholson's (1981) study of post-1974 TAA recipients addressed the principal deficiencies associated with Neumann's study. Although they did not use a comparison group, they adjusted their earnings loss estimates to account for the earnings growth that workers might have received had they not lost their job. They made that adjustment by using the relationship between earnings growth and tenure in predisplacement jobs.[3] They found this adjustment increased men's earnings losses by 20 percent, but added little to their estimates of women's losses. Overall, Corson and Nicholson found that most post-1974 TAA recipients were recalled, but those who were not recalled had large earnings losses. During the first two years following separation, permanently displaced male and female TAA recipients had earnings losses ranging from 30 to 50 percent. Even in the third year following their layoff, this group's earnings losses still averaged more than 10 percent ($3,100 in 1978 dollars) annually.

In an effort to expand its knowledge of the costs of worker displacement, ILAB sponsored an in-depth study of the steel industry. The steel industry was an important case study of the relationship between trade liberalization and worker dislocation for several reasons. First, at the time this geographically concentrated industry was experiencing strong import competition; second, its workers enjoyed wages among the highest of any U.S. industry; third, its workforce had relatively little formal education; and finally, it enforced rigid internal promotion policies for most blue-collar jobs. These factors all suggested that worker displacement would be associated with substantial earnings losses.

This study resembled earlier case studies in its focus on a worst-case scenario, but differed sharply from those studies in its use of a large administrative data set and in its econometric methodology. In his study of displacement costs, Jacobson (1977) used the earnings records from the Social Security Administration's (SSA) Longitudinal Employer/Employee Data (LEED) file. These data provided information on the age, race, sex, firm, and earnings histories of 24,000 steel workers covering the years 1957 through 1971. As a result, the study used a much larger sample with substantially longer earnings histories than the ones used by either Neumann or Corson and Nicholson.

Jacobson measured earnings losses as the difference between the actual earnings of displaced workers and their predicted earnings had they not lost their job. He computed their predicted earnings by using a comparison group of nondisplaced steel workers. Using this group of workers, he was able to predict how the earnings of displaced workers would have grown had they remained employed in the steel industry. His procedure represented an improvement over Corson and Nicholson's experience adjustment, because it explicitly took into account how contemporaneous economic conditions affected the rate of earnings growth of nondisplaced workers.[4]

From his empirical analysis, Jacobson concluded that dislocated steel workers suffered large and long-lasting earnings reductions, and that both younger and older workers experienced these losses. For workers with three or more years of tenure, earnings averaged 65 percent less than would otherwise have been expected over the first two years following displacement, and 45 percent less over the third through fifth years. In addition, he also found the following: (1) Initial losses were especially large due to unemployment; (2) the frequency of unemployment fell after two years, but earnings losses remained large; and (3) the characteristics of the local labor market at the time of displacement had an important effect on the short- and long-term losses.

Subsequent ILAB studies examined the costs of displacement among a broader set of industries. In one study, Jacobson (1978) used the LEED data to examine how these costs varied among workers displaced from 11 industries ranging from automobiles to women's clothing. As shown by table 2.1, he found that earnings losses varied considerably among industries. For workers displaced from the automobile, steel, and meat packing industries, losses from the third through the sixth year averaged approximately 15 percent. By contrast, for displaced electronics and women's clothing workers, earnings losses averaged less than 5 percent.

One potential shortcoming of the LEED data that is shared by the Pennsylvania data used in our study is that the file identifies job changes, but not the reasons for those changes. Jacobson limited his displacement loss estimates to workers in counties where industry employment had declined. Nevertheless, some of the separators in Jacobson's sample may not have been displaced, but instead may have quit their previous job or been dismissed for cause. Jacobson estimated the rate of normal attrition by examining the separation rates of industries in counties where employment was not declining. When attrition is high, job leavers are more likely to have quit to take higher paying jobs. In contrast, when attrition is low, a larger share of job leavers may have departed due to health or other personal problems. For our purposes, therefore, another important finding in Jacobson's study was that earnings losses from displacement were the largest for workers from industries with low attrition. That finding is consistent with the contention that workers in these industries have many job-specific skills and receive wage premiums.[5]

In principle, failure to differentiate between quits and involuntary layoffs could seriously bias downward the estimates of earnings losses. In the course of his analysis, Jacobson found that attrition was most common among younger workers and workers near retirement age. But, attrition was relatively rare among high-tenure, prime-age workers. In high-wage industries, the rate for these workers averaged only between 1 and 2 percent a year. Because of the similarity between our Pennsylvania data and the LEED file, these findings influenced us to limit our study to high-tenure, prime-age workers.

Holen et al. (1981) used another approach to address the problem that administrative earnings data do not distinguish between voluntary and involuntary separations. They used Social Security administrative records for a sample of 9,500 workers who left 42 plants that closed in 1971 or 1972. Although their study focused on plant closings, and only analyzed the experiences of workers from a few plants, there was no doubt that workers in their sample were dislocated. One potential drawback of their study is that they did not use a comparison group of nondisplaced workers from firms that did not close. Instead, like Corson and Nicholson, they used preseparation earnings growth to estimate what these workers' earnings would have been had they not been displaced. As did Corson and Nicholson, they found that this adjustment was small for women but substantial for men, especially for younger men.

Like Jacobson, Holen et al. found that prime-age men and women experienced especially large earnings losses during the two years following their plants' closings. However, in the subsequent three years, earnings losses were still large, averaging 15 percent per year for workers displaced from automobile, chemical, and glass firms. In roughly half the cases studied, however, losses became negligible or even became gains. Only among workers displaced from automobile

Table 2.1 Earnings Losses of Displaced Prime-Age Male Workers as Reported by Jacobson and Holen et al.

Industry	Average predisplacement earnings of sample (1980 dollars)	"Eleven-industry study"[a]		"Plant closing study"[b]	
		First two years	Subsequent four years	First two years	Subsequent three years
1. Automobiles	$15,918	43.4	15.6	24.1	14.6
2. Steel	15,175	43.6	12.6	—	—
3. Meat packing	14,133	23.9	18.1	—	—
4. Aerospace	18,947	23.6	14.8	—	—
5. Petrochemicals	18,498	12.4	12.5	15.9	16.4
6. Flat glass	16,291	—	—	16.3	12.2
7. Men's clothing	17,327	—	—	21.3	8.7
8. Women's clothing	12,406	13.3	2.1	—	—
9. Electronic components	17,433	8.3	4.1	10.1	0.2
10. Shoes	12,285	11.3	1.5	11.3	-1.9
11. Rubber footwear	15,322	—	—	32.2	-0.9
12. Toys	12,406	16.1	-2.7	—	—
13. TV receivers	15,605	0.7	-7.2	—	—
14. Cotton weaving	10,779	7.4	-11.4	7.6	5.2

a. Jacobson (1978) Loss estimates for industries 1-5 statistically significant at the 5 percent level. Negative sign indicates gains.
b. Holen, Jehn, and Trost (1981).

and chemicals firms did large losses persist throughout the sample period.[6]

Finally, one ILAB study addressed the question of earnings losses among displaced nonmanufacturing workers. In a study of displacement costs in two labor markets experiencing large employment declines, Jacobson (1984) found that losses during the first two years following displacement were large in both manufacturing and high-wage service industries such as finance, education, and health. Substantial losses persisted in manufacturing, education, and health services. These results indicate that even workers in non-trade-sensitive industries may be adversely affected by job loss. The results also indicate that low attrition was associated with large losses across sectors, reinforcing his earlier conclusion for manufacturing industries. Finally, predisplacement earnings and losses were substantially greater in almost every industry in Buffalo than in Providence. This result suggests that local labor market conditions are of considerable importance in assessing the likely magnitude of displaced worker earnings losses.

Taken together, the ILAB studies indicate that both men and women displaced from a variety of industries experienced significant earnings losses. However, the evidence also indicates that in some industries displacement need not be associated with large losses for the average displaced worker. Although most studies found substantial losses through the first two years, the findings on long-term losses are mixed, with some studies finding evidence of recovery in subsequent years. Workers seem most adversely affected if they were displaced from trade-sensitive durable goods industries where attrition rates were low.

2.3 Studies Using the Dislocated Worker Surveys

The ILAB-sponsored studies differed from the more recent dislocation literature. Because ILAB needed information to make decisions about modifying trade barriers on specific goods, there was a natural tendency to focus on how losses varied among industries rather than how they varied among different demographic groups. That interest in turn shaped the selection of data sets that were well-suited to study losses in particular industries. The LEED data and other administrative data sets provided researchers with exceptionally large samples of job separators' earnings histories. These samples permitted disaggregated industry analysis of the long-term costs of worker dislocation.

The ILAB data sets were, however, less than ideal for analyzing how losses varied according to worker characteristics, such as education, occupation, ethnicity, or marital status. Another problem with the data used in ILAB studies was that they were expensive to assemble. The U.S. Department of Labor incurred large expenses in developing several unique data sets. This expense was most obvious for the TAA surveys used by Neumann (1978a, 1978b) and by Corson and Nicholson (1981), and for the SSA data used in Holen and her colleagues' plant closing study. In addition, passage of the Tax Reform Act of 1976 made subsequent use of SSA data expensive and cumbersome by precluding dissemination of individual work histories.

The ILAB-sponsored studies showed that worker dislocation was often associated with substantial earnings losses. However, because these studies focused on the experiences of TAA recipients or of workers from particular industries or cities, little was known about how often workers were displaced. Accordingly, the Bureau of Labor Statistics designed the Displaced Worker Survey to count all workers who lost a job between 1979 and 1983.

Although the 1984 DWS and subsequent surveys also were expensive to conduct, they became public use data sets that researchers utilized in numerous studies. As a result, these studies have not only addressed the particular questions posed by policymakers, but also have examined more theoretical topics of interest to academic researchers. Among the questions of key interest to both groups has been (1) the characteristics of displaced workers; (2) the reemployment prospects and earnings losses of displaced workers; and (3) the factors that make job loss costly. In addition, academic researchers have extensively examined the link between the returns to job tenure and earnings losses.

Flaim and Seghal (1985) used the DWS to provide a clearer picture of the number and characteristics of displaced workers. The January 1984 version of this survey revealed that 13.9 million adult workers had lost a job between 1979 and 1983 because of "plant closings, employers going out of business, or layoffs from which they were not recalled." Flaim and Seghal argue that most of these job losers did not conform to the "general consensus as to who is and who is not a displaced worker." Such workers are generally regarded as having "spent many years in relatively high-paying jobs." The authors note that only 5.1 million of these workers had been employed three or more years at the time of their job loss (Flaim and Seghal 1985, p. 4).

As shown by table 2.2, these displaced workers were substantially more likely to have been males employed in manufacturing, in the Midwest, and in semiskilled and unskilled occupations than the rest of the labor force. Notably, only 60 percent of these workers were employed in January 1984. These employment rates were slightly lower among manufacturing, female, and unskilled workers, whereas the rates were higher among males, managers, and service workers.

Among those reemployed at the survey date, Flaim and Seghal found that earnings losses, as measured by the difference between their post- and predisplacement weekly earnings, varied considerably depending on their predisplacement industry. Losses of workers in durable goods averaged more than 20 percent. By contrast, the losses of workers in nondurable goods averaged less than 4 percent. These findings were consistent with those in some of the ILAB studies.

There are several reasons why it is difficult to interpret Flaim and Seghal's earnings loss estimates. First, as in Neumann's (1978b) TAA study, these estimates do not take into account the amount of time between job separations and the survey date. We have no way of knowing, therefore, whether these losses represent long-term setbacks. Second, the estimates are not adjusted for inflation. Because inflation was at a postwar high during the period, the real earnings losses may be substantially larger than indicated by the nominal losses. Finally, the figures do not account for how the earnings of those workers would have grown had they not lost their former job. Indeed, one shortcoming of many DWS studies is that they lack a comparison group to compute this growth.

Kosters (1986) addressed two of these issues by controlling for workers' year of displacement and the inflation rate. His main finding was that long-term losses among respondents in the DWS averaged about 20 percent in durable manufacturing and mining, but only about 7 percent in the other major industry groups. This finding led him to conclude that "... the costs of displacement apparently did not take the form of major widespread reductions in earnings. Instead, the main

Table 2.2 Characteristics of Displaced Workers: 1984 DWS Respondents with Three or More Years of Tenure

Characteristic	Percent of total labor force	Percent of displaced	Percent of DWS respondents employed on survey date	Percent of DWS respondents unemployed on survey date
Sex				
Male	56	65	64	27
Female	44	35	53	23
Race/Ethnicity[a]				
Black	9	12	42	41
Hispanic	5	6	52	34
White	88	86	63	23
Industry				
Manufacturing	20	49	60	26
Other goods producing	10	13	59	27
Transportation, communications, public utilities	7	7	58	27
Trade and services	63	31	64	21
Occupation				
Managers/professionals	23	14	75	17
Technical, sales, support	31	23	61	21
Services	14	5	51	24
Precision craft and repair	12	20	62	26

Characteristic	Percent of total labor force	Percent of displaced	Percent of DWS respondents employed on survey date	Percent of DWS respondents unemployed on survey date
Operators and laborers	16	36	55	32
Region				
New England	6	5	66	18
Mid-Atlantic	15	16	54	28
East North Central	17	24	51	33
West North Central	8	8	65	23
South Atlantic	17	13	69	18
East South Central	6	7	55	30
West South Central	11	10	71	18
Mountain	5	4	70	16
Pacific	15	13	60	27

SOURCES: Column 1: Handbook of Labor Statistics, U.S. Department of Labor, Bulletin 2217, June 1985, tables 2, 8, 15, 18, 19, and 43; pp. 8, 9, 26, 27, 41, 42, 49-55, and 96. Columns 2-4: Flaim and Seghal (1985), tables 1, 2, 3, and 4; pp. 4, 5, 7, and 8.

a. Categories are not mutually exclusive.

impact on economic well-being seems to have been some unemployment for most workers, extended periods of unemployment for a considerable portion of displaced workers, and eventually withdrawal from the work force of only a relatively small component" (p. 276).

Kosters' conclusions were generally consistent with those of Podgursky and Swaim (1987), who emphasize that a "substantial minority of workers experienced large and enduring losses" (pp. 21, 27). More than 30 percent of the reemployed full-time blue-collar workers and nearly 25 percent of reemployed full-time white-collar and service workers received wages that were more than 25 percent below their predisplacement levels.

As with many other DWS-based studies, a shortcoming of Kosters' study is that he did not use a comparison group. As seen in some of the ILAB studies, without a comparison group pre- versus postdisplacement earnings comparisons tend to substantially underestimate those losses for younger workers, whose real wages tend to grow rapidly with experience. Similarly, such comparisons tend to overestimate the losses for older workers whose real wages sometimes decline with experience.

Seitchik and Zornitsky (1989) conducted one of the few DWS studies that attempted to use a comparison group when measuring earnings losses. Their methodology differed from that used in many of the ILAB studies, because they drew their sample of nondisplaced workers from the Current Population Survey (CPS). However, the CPS data do not usually contain measures of respondents' tenure or previous wages. As a result, Seitchik and Zornitsky could not measure how earnings of these workers grew over time. Instead, they measured the costs of displacement as the regression adjusted difference between displaced and nondisplaced workers' wages. This regression adjustment took into account several differences between the two groups' characteristics, besides displacement status, that might cause their wages to differ.

Using this strategy, Seitchik and Zornitsky found that, on average, wages of displaced workers were 19 percent lower than those of their nondisplaced counterparts. However, the size of this gap depended on how long it had been since workers had lost their job. In the first year following a job loss, wages were nearly 30 percent less than those of nondisplaced workers. But by the fifth year after job loss, the gap had dropped to about 10 percent. This result suggests that earnings of displaced workers approach what they would have been had the worker not been displaced, not just that earnings approach their prejob loss levels. Indeed, as Kosters assumed, the findings of Seitchik and Zornitsky suggest that most workers had large initial losses that greatly diminished over time.[7] Finally, because their findings were similar to other DWS studies, their results suggest that when measuring long-run effects of displacement, it may not matter whether researchers use a comparison group.[8]

The accuracy of these conclusions is in doubt because of two key shortcomings in Seitchik and Zornitsky's study. First, their analysis used both low- and high-tenure displaced workers. Unlike Flaim and Seghal, they did not define displaced workers as job losers with three or more years of tenure. It might be the case that the recovery is complete for low-tenure workers, while high-tenure workers are left with large permanent declines. Indeed, Topel (1990, pp. 197, 205) found that long-term losses were as large as 40 percent for persons with 20 or more years of tenure. As a result, because Seitchik and Zornitsky did not control for tenure at the time of job loss, we cannot tell whether this hypothesis explains their findings.[9]

The more important potential problem with Seitchik and Zornitsky's empirical strategy is that the estimated wage losses may confound the consequences of worker displacement with differences between unobserved characteristics of displaced and nondisplaced workers. Their regression adjustment took into account only observable differences between these groups' characteristics. However, besides differences between observable characteristics, differences in hard-to-quantify characteristics such as quality of education or motivation might also cause wages of the two groups to be different.

One way to test whether the inability to control for unobserved characteristics affects Seitchik and Zornitsky's displacement cost estimates would be to compare the regression-adjusted predisplacement wages of displaced workers to those of a sample of nondisplaced workers. This sample of nondisplaced workers would not be the same as the one used in the postdisplacement period, but would include persons from several previous CPS files. Therefore, this test requires only several cross-sectional data sets and not longitudinal data. If there are no differences between displaced and nondisplaced workers' regression-adjusted predisplacement earnings, the regression-adjusted difference between the groups' postdisplacement earnings might reasonably represent the costs of displacement.

Although in principle this strategy can help validate Seitchik and Zornitsky's methodology, a recent study by Di la Rica (1992) indicates that in practice it may not be successful. When she compared the regression-adjusted predisplacement wages of the 1986 DWS respondents to those of a comparison group drawn from the CPS, she found that the displaced workers' wages were lower. This predisplacement wage gap is consistent with the notion that wages of displaced workers decline during the periods leading up to their job losses. However, it is also consistent with the view that displaced and nondisplaced workers have different unobserved characteristics and that these differences account for the gap between their postdisplacement wages. Under either interpretation, Seitchik and Zornitsky's methodology cannot be validated with the DWS predisplacement wage data.

Madden (1988) developed an alternative comparison group for her DWS study by constructing longitudinal data from the CPS files. Because some respondents to the January 1984 CPS also responded to the January 1983 survey, she was able to construct a sample of displaced and nondisplaced workers whose wages she observed in 1983 and 1984.[10] She could compare the wage change of those displaced during that period to that of comparable nondisplaced workers. An advantage of this approach is that it explicitly takes into account how earnings of displaced workers would have grown had they not been displaced. Further, by comparing differences in wage growth between the two groups, the approach implicitly takes into account fixed unobservable characteristics that might affect workers' wages.

As Swaim and Podgursky (1991) note in their critique of Madden's study, average wage loss estimates rise by as much as 50 percent when a comparison group is used in the analysis.[11] They observe, however, that several problems with Madden's strategy make it difficult in practice to determine how important it is to use a comparison group when estimating earnings losses. Among the most important problems is Madden's small sample size. After matching the CPS in successive years, she was left with only 143 displaced males and 65 displaced females. Further, she was only able to examine the wage effects of displacement for workers who had been displaced for less than one year, when differences might be greatest anyway. Finally, many of the workers dislocated in the year closest to the interview date may have been recalled subsequently. Thus, that sample is not representative of workers certain to be permanently displaced. As a result of these problems, matched-CPS samples are not likely to lead to improved studies of worker displacement.

2.4 Earnings Losses and the Returns to Tenure

Much academic research on displacement has examined whether human capital theory can account for the observed earnings reductions following dislocation. Those studies usually compare the estimated returns to tenure and to experience (age minus years of education minus 6) before and after workers involuntarily separate from jobs. The underlying assumption in these studies is that tenure measures specific skills that are not easily transferred from one job to the next, whereas experience measures general skills that workers take with them when they separate from their firms.

The advantage of these assumptions is that they yield a relatively straightforward way of predicting the magnitude of displacement costs. As Hamermesh (1987) and others have argued, when workers involuntarily separate from their firms they lose the returns from tenure. Thus, it is predicted that their starting wages on their new job should depend only on years of experience, education, and other non-firm-specific characteristics. This framework yields a relatively simple way to compute earnings losses associated with displacement. To see how to make these calculations, consider the following wage equation:

(2.1) $\log(w_i) = x_i\beta + 0.018*\text{tenure} - 0.0004*\text{tenure squared}$,

where $\log(w_i)$ denotes a worker's natural log wages, x_i denotes years of experience and other non-firm-specific characteristics, and tenure refers to years of service at the firm (see Hamermesh 1987, p. 63). Based on the foregoing assumptions, the predicted starting wage for workers who involuntarily separate from their firms is $x_i\beta$. Therefore, workers' wage losses simply depend on their tenure. Based on equation (2.1), we predict that the wages of a worker with 10 years of tenure would decline by 14 percent, whereas for a worker with 20 years of tenure they would decline by 20 percent.[12]

The advantage of this approach is that estimates of displacement's cost may be derived from studies of the returns to tenure on the job. While the magnitude of these returns is not yet completely settled, other studies provide policymakers with estimates of these returns that are of similar magnitude to that given in equation (2.1). For example, Topel (1991) finds in the Panel Study of Income Dynamics (PSID) that 10 years of tenure is associated with a 25 percent increase in wages. Therefore, he would predict that when such workers are displaced, their wages would be 25 percent lower on their postdisplacement jobs. Most important, if researchers and policymakers can estimate displacement costs from existing research, they do not require costly and specialized surveys or data sets such as the DWS or LEED.

As appealing as the foregoing approach may be, it is likely to produce misleading estimates of the costs of displacement when using a cross-sectional data set like the DWS. This finding does not refute the human capital framework, but instead indicates the difficulties surrounding attempts to estimate the returns to tenure and to predict who is likely to be displaced. Addison and Portugal (1989) and others argue that unobserved characteristics arc correlated with tenure. This relation implies that high-tenure workers earn more than low-tenure workers, in part because they have more general skills. Indeed, they found that tenure on a worker's predisplacement job is associated with higher earnings on the postdisplacement job.

Addison and Portugal concluded that their "empirical results together provide a strong indictment of approaches that, in computing earnings losses, focus on estimates of the loss of firm-specific human capital investments obtained from the coefficient on tenure in a predisplacement wage equation. While there may indeed be significant losses associated with yet to be fully depreciated specific training investments (some hint as to which may be provided by the strongly negative coefficients associated with change in industry and occupation), the extent of such losses cannot be gauged from the tenure coefficient since the latter compounds a number of different effects" (p. 297). The upshot of Addison and Portugal's study was that in order to estimate the losses associated with worker displacement, researchers require information on workers' job changes, including their earnings before and after job loss.

Kletzer (1990) used the empirical framework just described to generate separate estimates of the effects of tenure and experience on the earnings and earnings losses of displaced blue- and white-collar men and women. As shown by table 2.3, prior to dislocation, the returns to tenure were larger for white-collar than for blue-collar workers and larger for women than for men. At the same time, the returns to experience (as proxied by age) were larger for white-collar workers and men than they were for blue-collar workers and women. These findings were generally consistent with those in the existing human capital literature.

Like Addison and Portugal, Kletzer also found that predislocation tenure remained an important determinant of postdisplacement earnings. More significant, however, she found that the importance of predisplacement tenure varied considerably among the groups studied. As shown by table 2.3, blue-collar men's and white-collar women's earnings rose only one-half as fast with predisplacement tenure after dislocation as they had prior to dislocation. By contrast, the effect of tenure on earnings was much more similar in the two periods for blue-collar women and white-collar men.

As shown by rows 5 and 6 of table 2.3, the foregoing findings imply that for some groups earnings losses vary substantially with predisplacement tenure, while for other groups tenure is not an important determinant of earnings losses. Kletzer's estimates imply that a blue-collar man displaced after 15 years of service has losses that are 13 percent larger than those of a similar worker displaced after only five years on the job. However, a blue-collar woman with 15 years of service has losses that are actually 2 percent less than her counterpart with five years of tenure.

These findings for blue-collar women indicate how poor an indicator estimates of the returns to predisplacement tenure may be for predicting the costs of worker dislocation. As shown in rows 3 and 4 of table 2.3, this group had the largest returns to tenure. Yet, as suggested in rows 1 and 2, these women were able to transport most of the skills associated with that tenure to their new job. Therefore, tenure was a poor predictor of their earnings losses.

Table 2.3 The Effect of Predisplacement Tenure on Earnings: Coefficients on Tenure from Earnings Regressions

Effect on log earnings	Blue-collar		White-collar	
	Men	Women	Men	Women
Postdisplacement earnings				
Predisplacement tenure	.016	.028	.020	.022
Predisplacement tenure squared/100	-.077	-.103	-.075	-.098
Predisplacement earnings				
Predisplacement tenure	.030	.032	.026	.039
Predisplacement tenure squared/100	-.080	-.072	-.071	-.135
Difference between postdisplacement and predisplacement earnings				
Predisplacement tenure	-.014	-.004	-.008	-.017
Predisplacement tenure squared/100	.003	-.031	-.004	.037

SOURCE: Kletzer (1991), tables 3-6 and A-1, pp. 116-19, 129.
NOTE: The figures in the table are the coefficients on tenure and tenure squared in predisplacement job from a regression of log weekly earnings on individual characteristics. Other independent variables include age, education, race, marital status, occupation, industry, and part-time status.

Taken together, the DWS studies usually point to larger earnings losses as predisplacement tenure increases. Kletzer's (1991) study makes clear, however, that there are important exceptions to this finding. As indicated by table 2.3, even among men this finding depends on whether we are examining the experience of blue-collar or white-collar males. This caveat is important for our empirical work in the following chapters. We are inclined to believe that because we focus our analysis on the experiences of high-tenure displaced workers, the losses we observe are larger than for the average worker who involuntarily loses his or her job. But, as Kletzer's study indicates, we cannot be sure that some groups of workers with less tenure do not have losses that are just as large.

The findings from the DWS studies on the relationship between experience and earnings losses are somewhat more clear-cut than those on the relationship between tenure and earnings losses. On the whole, the findings suggest that as long as we compare workers with similar years of service on their predisplacement job, earnings losses will rise only modestly with years of experience or age. For example, Topel finds that men's earnings losses rise by 1/2 percent for each year of prior labor market experience (1990, table 8, p. 203). Likewise, Kletzer's estimates of male wage losses are comparable to Topel's (1991, tables 3-6, pp. 116-19, and appendix A-1, p. 129). The earnings losses for workers with similar years of service are about 10 percentage points larger for displaced 50-year-olds than they are for displaced 30-year-olds. Among women the differences in losses are smaller than among men, with some evidence that older white-collar women have smaller earnings losses than do their younger counterparts. Finally, Addison and Portugal use a richer empirical specification and find that once they control for tenure, there is little evidence that displaced men's earnings losses vary significantly with years of experience, except for those workers over 50.[13]

2.5 The Advantages of Using Longitudinal Data

The foregoing DWS studies have several shortcomings that can potentially be addressed with longitudinal data sets such as the PSID or those based on administrative records. First, the DWS data on layoffs and predisplacement wages are from retrospective interviews. In contrast, longitudinal data is collected by survey takers revisiting the household each period. Therefore, longitudinal data are less likely to be tainted by recall bias, in which workers either forget past layoffs or report that the layoff occurred more recently than the actual date. Topel (1990) finds evidence that respondents in the CPS tended to forget events far in the past, especially those that likely involved small wage losses. As a result, data sets like the DWS "will substantially understate the total amount of worker displacement that actually occurred over the period in question and also will misestimate the timing of events" (p. 190).

A second shortcoming of DWS-based studies is that as with any cross-sectional data set, it is difficult to distinguish between the long-term effects of displacement and the effects of being displaced during poor economic conditions. For example, in the 1984 DWS, workers displaced five years before the survey were displaced in 1979. However, there is no way to know whether long-term estimates of wage losses result (1) from displacement, (2) from the consequences of being displaced in 1979, or (3) from deteriorating economic conditions that caused average earnings levels to decline. By contrast, Topel's study using the PSID employs a panel of workers displaced between 1968 and 1985. As a result, he can distinguish between the effects of changing labor market conditions and of elapsed time since displacement.

The importance of these issues is heightened because findings based on the PSID appear to differ from those based on the DWS. Topel found in both the DWS and the PSID that four years after their displacements, blue-collar manufacturing workers had wages 20 percent below their predisplacement levels. But, among nonmanufacturing workers, losses were much larger among workers in the DWS than those in the PSID. More important, his findings on the importance of tenure and experience differed substantially between the two data sets. In the DWS he found, as had others, that predisplacement tenure was a better predictor of losses than was experience. However, when he used the PSID, he found that the losses did not rise even modestly with tenure, yet rose dramatically with years of labor market experience. According to his PSID estimates, a 50-year-old displaced blue-collar worker's losses were approximately 33 percent larger than the losses for a comparable 30-year-old (Topel 1990, p. 203). This finding is puzzling. As Topel noted, "it would seem that the duration of employment with a single firm is a better indicator of the degree of specialization in a worker's skills. Yet tenure has no long-run effect (on losses) in the (PSID) data, while total market experience does" (Topel 1990, pp. 204-6).

A third shortcoming of DWS-based studies is that they often fail to employ a comparison group. Further, as we observed above, even when they use a comparison group it is usually under less than ideal circumstances. By contrast, studies based on a data set like the PSID may use the earnings histories of nondisplaced workers to estimate how earnings of displaced workers would have grown had they not lost their job. In one such study Ruhm (1991b) finds that workers displaced between 1971 and 1975 experience long-term wage losses that amount to between 11 and 14 percent of their expected earnings (pp. 174-75). Ruhm argues that these losses depend on the use of a comparison group, because displaced workers "missed out entirely on the 8.4 percent real wage gain obtained by the control group over the same period" (Ruhm 1991a, pp. 320-21).

To see how important the use of a comparison group may be to studies of the cost of worker dislocation, consider Topel's analysis of displaced workers from the PSID. He did not use a comparison group of nondisplaced workers to measure how earnings of displaced workers might have grown had they not lost their job. Without a comparison group, he found that earnings losses as measured by the difference between post- and predisplacement earnings did not vary by tenure. But because nondisplaced workers with low tenure are likely to have faster earnings growth than are high-tenure workers, those low-tenure workers might have "missed out" on some substantial earnings growth. As a result, had Topel used a comparison group he might have found a counterintuitive negative relationship between tenure and earnings losses.

A final shortcoming of DWS-based studies is that they use reported "usual" weekly earnings of workers at the time of job loss. However, if wages and hours decline in the periods prior to displacement, DWS measures of earnings losses will understate the losses associated with the events that lead to job separations. For example, if the initial response of firms to changing economic conditions or policies is to reduce hours or real wages, earnings and wages will fall prior to job loss. As we argue in subsequent chapters, these earnings declines represent a significant portion of displaced worker earnings losses. Indeed, Ruhm (1991b), using the PSID, finds that the losses during these years may amount to as much as 60 percent of the long-term losses of workers (pp. 169, 175-76).

Despite the merits of using longitudinal data sets such as the PSID to estimate the costs of worker dislocation, there are also some drawbacks. First, the sample sizes of the PSID or the National Longitudinal Surveys are relatively small. Topel notes that "only 1400 displacement 'events' are derivable from the panel, and of these only 120 involve long-term jobs that lasted ten years or more" (1990, p. 184). A second drawback is that people drop out of the sample with time. If those who leave the sample are more likely to have been displaced, estimates of losses are likely to be biased. A third drawback is that the PSID does not distinguish between layoff and discharges for cause. A worker who has been fired would be expected to have lower subsequent earnings, but for reasons that are different from those of a worker laid off for economic reasons. Finally, even in data sets like the PSID, displacement events and earnings are self-reported. While the problems with self-reporting are likely to be less severe in surveys where respondents are interviewed repeatedly than in surveys like the DWS, errors may arise that would not appear in data sets that use administrative records.

2.6 Summary

The previous literature provides abundant evidence that worker displacement leads to substantial earnings losses. This literature consistently reports increased frequencies of unemployment and corresponding large earnings losses during the two years following job separations. There is also consensus on the importance of some worker characteristics in determining the magnitude of these losses. For example, most studies find that gender is not a very important predictor of earnings losses, as neither men nor women are immune to repercussions of displacement. At the same time, these studies find that depressed local labor market conditions increase workers' losses.

There is less consensus in the literature about whether these losses persist and how important are age, tenure on the predisplacement job, and former industry in determining the size of the losses. Some studies report long-term losses averaging 15 to 20 percent per year or more, while others argue that the long-term losses are substantially smaller. Some studies argue that these losses are limited to workers from trade-sensitive durable goods industries, while others find more widespread losses. Finally, some studies assert that tenure is an important predictor of worker losses, while others find that tenure is only modestly important and instead that age has a larger impact on their subsequent earnings.

In light of the different methodological approaches and data sets that have been used in the literature, the lack of consensus surrounding some questions on the earnings impact of worker displacement is not surprising. The main problem, of course, is that none of the data sets used in these analyses have been ideal, and that data deficiencies have in large part dictated methodological approaches seen in the literature. The LEED or SSA administrative data have long earnings histories and information on their industry, but little information on workers characteristics. The DWS provides the clearest picture of displaced worker characteristics, but has limited earnings histories and is plagued by respondent recall bias. The PSID has both long earnings histories and abundant information on worker characteristics, but the sample size of displaced workers is relatively small, especially the numbers of high-tenure job losers.

Although the data used in our study are by no means ideal, one purpose of this monograph is to show how state administrative data can contribute to the literature on worker dislocation. The long quarterly earnings histories available for large numbers of workers enables us to generate a clearer picture of the temporal pattern of earnings losses and to evaluate a wider variety of alternative hypotheses, besides job losses, that might account for the lower earnings experienced by displaced workers. In the following chapter we show how state administrative data can be prepared and used in an analysis of the costs of worker dislocation.

NOTES

1. Currently, eligibility for extended UI benefits under TAA requires meeting a three-part test: (1) employment in the worker's plant and industry must have fallen absolutely, (2) a petition must be filed and certified by the Department of Labor that the importation of goods that directly compete with that plant's production was at least partly responsible for the decline, and (3) the certified worker must have entered training (or received a waiver) prior to the 13th week of unemployment.

2. A disturbing finding from studies of the post-1974 TAA program was the large percentage of TAA recipients who were subsequently recalled to their former jobs. Because these workers were recalled, they experienced small earnings losses. The high recall rates and relatively short durations of unemployment differed sharply from the experiences of the pre-1974 TAA recipients. These results troubled policymakers because the legitimacy of the TAA program rested largely on the view that trade-impacted workers were absorbing unusually high costs and therefore merited special attention. As a result of the evidence that many TAA recipients were better off than workers whose displacement did not result from trade, Congress reduced TAA to the level of regular UI benefits.

3. To be more precise, they estimated the earnings growth that would have occurred by using the coefficients from a regression of predisplacement earnings on tenure. In the absence of displacement, they estimated that men's earnings would have grown by nearly 10 percent, and women's by less than 5 percent.

4. Operationally, he regressed both displaced and nondisplaced workers' earnings on age, tenure, race, and several years of predisplacement earnings. Those controls for prior earnings captured the effect of unobserved fixed characteristics on current earnings. Finally, to measure the earnings effect of displacement, he included a dummy variable indicating whether the worker had been displaced.

5. Jacobson also attempted to measure the change in earnings for workers who left jobs for nondisplacement-related reasons by comparing industry-specific earnings levels of workers in counties where industry employment rose or remained constant to counties where employment fell. The results showed that after a year or two, earnings changes were similar to those of displaced workers. This suggests that where attrition was low, few workers left to attain higher wages. Rather, voluntary leavers departed for noneconomic factors. At the same time, where attrition was high both displaced workers and other job leavers obtained similar jobs in the long run.

6. Holen et al. found that losses were frequently greater in percentage terms in the short run and more persistent for women than men. Women appeared to return to work more slowly than men, and had a greater likelihood of accepting part-time or part-year employment. Holen et al. also made a major effort to deal with problems stemming from the high incidence with which women left the labor force entirely. Difficulties in accurately measuring labor force status with administrative data influenced our decision to focus our study on workers who showed strong labor force attachment.

7. Analyses using SSA data showed substantial recoveries as well. But SSA-based studies examined annual earnings, not weekly earnings. The recovery of annual earnings is likely to be sharp because unemployment, which is especially great initially, is included in that measure.

8. Podgursky and Swaim (1987, p. 19) experimented with a similar strategy and found that median losses were "somewhat larger" when they used a comparison group.

9. Even though Seitchik and Zornitsky did not observe the tenure of their nondisplaced workers, they still could have examined its effects on the losses of displaced workers. One simple strategy would have been to follow Flaim and Seghal's definition and define displaced workers with

less than three years of tenure as low-tenure workers and those with three or more years of tenure as high-tenure workers. They then could have compared the regression-adjusted wages of these two groups to those of the nondisplaced workers. This strategy does not resolve the methodological concerns discussed below.

10. Because the Bureau of the Census altered the household codes in 1985, it is impossible to construct such a matched sample of displaced and nondisplaced workers from the 1986 DWS. However, matches are possible for the 1988 and 1990 surveys.

11. See Madden (1988, table 2, pp. 102-3). For reemployed males, Madden finds that postdisplacement 1984 wages are 9.5 percent below predisplacement wages. However, nondisplaced workers' wages grew by 4.3 percent between 1983 and 1984. Swaim and Podgursky (1991) assert that these percentages cannot be compared, because displaced workers' 1983 wages are not their January 1983 wages but their 1983 wages just prior to displacement.

12. We derive the 14 percent figure from ([0.018*10 - 0.0004*100]*100%) and the 20 percent figure from ([0.018*20 - 0.0004*400]*100%).

13. See Addison and Portugal (1989, pp. 288-89). Instead of examining the relationship between earnings losses and age, as did Topel, they examined the relationship between earnings losses and three linear splines for age. Their age categories were 20-35 years, 36-50 years, and 51-65 years.

3
The Use of Administrative Data in the Study of Worker Dislocation

In our introductory chapter, we argued that there are several reasons why earnings might decline when dislocated workers lose their jobs. In chapter 2, we reviewed a considerable literature indicating that involuntary job loss is costly. That literature indicates that at least during the first few years following job loss, earnings and wage rates remain significantly below their former levels. Still, disagreement continues about the magnitude and persistence of these losses. In this monograph, we show how state administrative records can contribute to the displacement literature by revealing the temporal pattern of displaced workers' earnings losses. In particular, because these data include long earnings histories for a large number of workers, they are well suited to estimating the long-term costs of worker dislocation and the rate at which earnings recover after workers secure new employment.

Accordingly, in this chapter we describe both the advantageous and disadvantageous features of our administrative data and highlight some of the conceptual problems that arise when using such data to estimate the cost of worker dislocation. In section 3.1, we explain how we constructed our sample and comment on some of its strengths and weaknesses. In section 3.2, we motivate our decision to focus on workers who demonstrated a high degree of attachment to the Pennsylvania wage and salary work force. In section 3.3, we compare the characteristics of our sample of separators to those of workers from the Displaced Workers Survey (DWS) and the Current Population Survey (CPS). Finally, in section 3.4, we discuss some of the potential statistical problems that arise when we use our administrative data and conventional estimators to estimate earnings losses of displaced workers.

3.1 The Pennsylvania Data

The statistical framework developed for this study applies generally to the problem of estimating earnings losses associated with worker dislocation. However, the empirical work reported here is limited to estimation of the losses suffered by displaced workers from Pennsylvania. We have restricted our attention to those workers in order to take advantage of an unusual data set that we have constructed by combining information from administrative sources on Pennsylvania workers and their firms. These sources provide us with a large sample of quarterly earnings histories extending from 1974 through 1986.

Although we cannot guarantee that our findings on earnings losses of displaced Pennsylvania workers are representative of all displaced worker experiences, it is worth noting that Pennsylvania is a large state with a diverse industrial base. Further, during the 1980s, the period covered by this study, the economic performance of the eastern half of the state was considerably different from that of the western half of the state. The state's southeastern section shared in the mid-1980s growth with the other middle Atlantic states and New England, while many areas in the western sections were mired in the double digit unemployment rates that were common in states bordering the Great Lakes.[1]

3.1.1 Constructing the Data

We constructed our longitudinal sample from state UI tax reports and ES202 reports of Pennsylvania firms that employed 50 or more workers in 1979. The UI tax records contain quarterly wage and salary reports from all Pennsylvania wage and salary sources.[2] We aggregated these reports to obtain the total quarterly earnings for a 5 percent sample of Pennsylvania workers.[3] For each calendar year, we designated the worker's principal employer as the firm from which he or she received the most earnings. We also retained the fraction of a worker's quarterly earnings paid by the principal employer. These earnings data should be relatively free of the kind of measurement error that plagues survey data. Because the state requires accurate and timely information to calculate firms' UI taxes and worker's benefits, it cross-checks the UI tax reports against earlier reports and federal corporate tax returns.

ES202 reports of firms provide information about their employment levels.[4] The state uses this information to calculate tax rates, particularly in multiplant firms. We created our longitudinal file by merging the information on quarterly earnings of workers with the ES202 records of their principal employers for each year. For each worker in the sample, we have information on quarterly earnings and, for each calendar year, the principal employer, SIC industry, location, and average employment during the last, current, and following years. Using that information we constructed employees' years of service with their employer back to 1974.

3.1.2 Identifying Job Changes

As we noted in chapter 2, the only way we can tell whether displacements are a major setback to workers' careers is by analyzing data on actual job changes. Therefore, a key element of our analysis is accurately tracking job separations from individual firms. Both the UI tax reports and ES202 data include Employer Identification Numbers (EIN) of firms. In principle, we can identify job changes by changes in the principal employers' EIN numbers. Unfortunately, in practice actual job changes are more difficult to identify. In several years, more than 5 percent of total employment was in firms where employees remained with a firm whose EIN number changed. Because firm EIN change is common, failure to correct for EIN changes would result in many bogus job changes. Indeed, had we not eliminated these bogus job changes, they would be the primary source of movement of workers between employers within the same 4-digit SIC industry.

Any change in a firm's legal structure triggers an EIN change. The four main sources of EIN changes are listed below in order of their frequency.

1. Reorganizations where a firm switches from one EIN to another

2. Takeovers and acquisitions where one firm switches to the EIN of a preexisting firm

3. Mergers where two or more firms switch to a new EIN

4. Spin-offs and divestitures where one firm continues to use its old EIN, but a portion of the firm begins to use a new EIN.

Because Pennsylvania wants to prevent firms from "running away" from their UI experience-rated tax rates, all EIN changes are tracked in successor-predecessor files. With these files in hand, we used a complex matching procedure to reassign the firms that changed, except for spin-offs, to the EIN used by the firm (or its successors) at the end of the sample period. Using a single EIN for each family of related firms ensures that workers who change EINs are actually changing firms. Of course, some workers may have moved between firms that at some other time were joined, but this must have been a rare occurrence. In addition, using a single EIN permitted employment changes to be accurately measured in years surrounding EIN changes. Because firms sometimes change their corporate structure when they reduce their workforces, these procedures were particularly crucial when we later created a subsample of workers who separated from firms that engaged in mass layoffs.

Unfortunately, accounting for recorded EIN changes would not necessarily capture all bogus job changes. In rare instances an EIN change might occur when a firm ceased operations and, without a formal sale, another firm acquired the plant and began operations with many of the same workers. To detect the occurrence of any such restarts and to check the accuracy of the successor-predecessor file, we isolated all EIN changes for which more than one worker in our sample moved from an old EIN to the same new EIN. Next, we checked whether the old EIN continued in use, or whether all workers reporting under the old EIN shifted to the new EIN. These checks demonstrated that the successor-predecessor file was accurate in linking old and new EINs, but was inaccurate when dating or distinguishing among the four types of EIN changes. In addition, we found no definite cases of restarts and less than 50 cases where the evidence that a restart occurred was ambiguous. (The ambiguity arose because the starting date and ending dates for EIN numbers on the ES202 forms were inaccurate.)

3.1.3   Dating Worker Separations

In order to investigate the temporal pattern of earnings losses associated with worker dislocation, we also had to identify the quarters in which employees separated from their firms. Our administrative data included two pieces of information that we could use to identify separation dates. First, a change in the principal employer's EIN number from one year to the next was taken as an indication that the worker had separated from the firm during one of the two years. Second, changes in the percentages of quarterly earnings received from a given year's principal employer signaled whether a job transition might have occurred during a particular quarter.

To date the precise quarter of separation, we determined the last quarter that the worker received earnings from the old principal employer. When this quarter was in the last year in which the old employer was still the principal employer, the quarter of separation was the last quarter of positive earnings from that firm. For example, if during the last year with the old principal employer, the worker received earnings from the old employer in the third, but not the fourth quarter, we designated the third quarter as the quarter of separation. However, when the employee received 100 percent of fourth quarter earnings from the old principal employer, the separation quarter was the last quarter of the following year in which the employee received earnings from sources other than the new principal employer (unless there were quarters of zero earnings). For example, if the worker received all of his or her earnings from the new principal employer in the second but not the first quarter, we designated the first quarter as the quarter of separation.

In most instances the foregoing procedure precisely dates the separation. But there appear to be two exceptional cases: first, when the employee has another wage or salary job besides the job with the old principal employer; and second, when the old principal employer grants the employee severance pay after displacement. Both of those exceptions may cause us to date the separation after it actually occurred. As a result of our dating procedure, some earnings may falsely appear to decline during the quarters prior to displacement. We investigate the potential importance of this possibility in chapter 5.

3.1.4   Addressing the Shortcomings of State Administrative Records

Despite our efforts, our administrative data set has two principal disadvantages compared with other data sets used in the displacement literature. First, the only available demographic characteristics of workers are year of birth, sex, and tenure with their firms since 1974. By comparison, other data sets, such as the DWS or the PSID, include a wider array of characteristics—among them educational attainments, occupations, and marital or union status. The reason we even have information on age and sex is that the State of Pennsylvania obtained these data in 1976 from the Social Security Administration (SSA).[5] As a result, we have these demographics only for persons employed in that year in wage and salary jobs for whom the SSA could match the state's records to their own records of last names and Social Security numbers. Therefore, unlike other dislocation studies, we cannot learn how workers' losses vary by their educational attainments, occupation, or marital or union status. However, we do not view this lack of demographics as an important shortcoming of our analysis. As we show in chapters 5 and 6, we can still provide an extensive picture on how their losses vary with time according to sex, age, industry, and region of the state.

A second disadvantage of our data is they do not directly identify whether job separations are quits, discharges for cause, or layoffs due to economic difficulties of firms. As a result, our displaced worker sample may include some workers who left their former jobs because they either quit or were discharged for cause. This second shortcoming is clearly more important than the first. Although other data sets do not distinguish between discharges for cause and layoffs, they do try to distinguish between quits and layoffs. They are right to do this because the literature indicates that quits and layoffs represent employment separations under different economic circumstances (e.g., McLaughlin 1991). One thing that these differing circumstances entail is that persons who quit their jobs are less likely to experience earnings losses than persons who are laid off. Because, in effect, we mix displaced workers with those who quit their jobs, our earnings loss estimates may tend to understate the costs of worker dislocation.

The importance of not being able to distinguish between quits and layoffs is reduced in our study because it focuses on the experiences of high-tenure, prime-age displaced workers. In chapters 5 and 6, we examine the earnings histories of workers who were born between 1930 and 1959 and who had the same principal employer from 1974 through the end of 1979 before separating from their firms between 1980 and 1986. Because our sample includes only persons who worked for the same firm during the 1970s, they all had six or more years of tenure when they separated from their firms. Further, because every one in the sample was born after 1930, none of the separators was near normal retirement age. These workers are much less likely than low-tenure workers or older workers to leave their firms voluntarily.

Despite the stated shortcomings, our administrative data have several advantages over other data sets used in the dislocation literature. These advantages derive from the large sample of 13-year quarterly earnings histories and from the merging of these histories to information about firms. The sample that we analyze in chapters 5 and 6 of high-tenure separators who remain attached to Pennsylvania's workforce includes over 9,507 persons who separated from 2,484 different firms. By comparison to other longitudinal data sets, the number of observations in this sample is approximately the same as the number of household heads in the PSID and far exceeds the number of "displaced" workers in that data set. In addition, we also have a sample of nearly 14,000 similarly tenured nondisplaced workers whose earnings we can use to identify the likely path that earnings of displaced workers might have taken had they not lost their jobs.

Besides its large size, our data set also includes information on firms, such as their employment levels and changes, their geographical location, and their 4-digit SIC industry. One benefit of this information is that we do not have to rely on retrospective interviews to determine when workers separated from their firms and how much they "usually" made prior to their separations. In the DWS, respondents were asked about job losses that had occurred as long as five years prior to their interviews. In our study, we rely on quarterly tax reports of firms to identify job changes.

Another benefit of knowing employment levels of firms is that we can identify individuals who separated from firms that have experienced a substantial reduction in their workforces or even a complete closing. These workers are less likely than other job separators to be leaving because they quit or as a result of their own poor job performance. In chapter 6 we examine the earnings histories of a subsample of workers who separated from firms whose employment had fallen by more than 30 percent from its 1970s levels. Yet despite this sample restriction we are still left with a sample of 6,435 workers separating from 1,537 different firms.

3.2   Choosing Among Alternative Samples of Separators

Relatively simple tabulations of the Pennsylvania data indicate that displaced workers experience substantial long-term earnings losses. Figure 3.1 shows that the earnings[6] of a subset of our sample of high-tenure workers—those who separated from their firms during the first quarter of 1982—fell sharply after they left their former firms.[7] More important, in 1986, four years after their separations, these workers' earnings were still nearly $4,000 per quarter less than employees with similar tenure who remained at their firms. It is unlikely that the post-separation earnings differences result from preexisting differences between the productivity and skills of the two groups. As the figure indicates, during the mid-1970s, the earnings of workers who subsequently separated from their firms were nearly the same as for those who stayed at their firms.

The earnings losses depicted in figure 3.1 correspond to declines of well over 50 percent of the affected workers' predisplacement earnings and could easily be described as catastrophic. However, caution is needed in interpreting those results. Figure 3.2 shows, for each quarter, the fraction of workers in the two groups who have positive earnings from Pennsylvania wage and salary employment. Evidently, the fraction of separators with positive earnings drops dramatically after they leave their former firms and remains at low levels for the rest of the sample period.[8] Unfortunately, it is not possible to determine from state administrative records whether workers without Pennsylvania earnings are genuinely unemployed, have retired, have become self-employed, have moved out of the state, or are working under another Social Security number.

Figure 3.1 Quarterly Earnings (1987$) of Workers Separating in Quarter 82.I and Workers Staying Through Quarter 86.IV

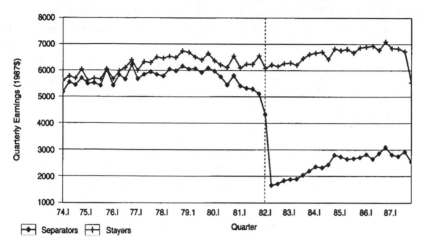

Figure 3.2 Quarterly Employment Rates of Workers Separating in Quarter 82.I and Workers Staying Through Quarter 86.IV

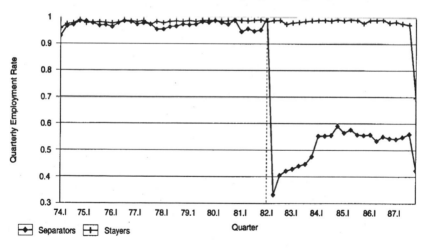

Our inability to distinguish among these possible reasons for a worker having zero quarterly earnings complicates our analysis of displaced worker earnings losses. Among those workers who are unemployed, a record with zero earnings is accurate. However, when we assume that the other groups have or would have zero earnings, we clearly overstate the losses associated with displacement. For example, if retired persons reentered the labor market, most would find jobs. Similarly, the self-employed, those who left the state, and those working under a different Social Security number probably have positive earnings.

In order to mitigate the problems associated with earnings records of these workers, we have chosen to further restrict our analyses to workers who demonstrate a high degree of attachment to the Pennsylvania wage and salary workforce.[9] Specifically, we require that workers have positive earnings in every calendar year between 1974 and 1986. This restriction clearly resolves the interpretative difficulties associated with persons who leave the state following their job losses. But it does exclude from our sample all workers who were unemployed continuously for two or more years following their displacements.[10] Figure 3.3 shows how the earnings of this high-attachment group of workers evolve after they separate from their firms in the first quarter of 1982. As the figure shows, this groups' 1986 earnings were $2,000 per quarter, or 20 percent below those of workers who stayed with their firms through the end of 1986. While still very significant, that earnings difference is only half the size of the earnings difference for the full sample of workers separating in the first quarter of 1982.

Figure 3.3 Quarterly Earnings (1987$) of High-Attachment Workers Separating in Quarter 82.I and Workers Staying Through Quarter 86.IV

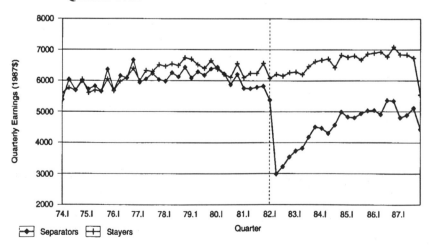

3.3 The Representativeness of Our Sample

We recognize that because of the way we constructed our sample, our empirical findings on displaced worker earnings losses may not be representative of the losses experienced by workers without high labor force attachment or by those displaced workers who left Pennsylvania. However, a comparison between the characteristics of our sample and those of workers never having positive wage or salary earnings in Pennsylvania after they separate from their firms suggests that the two samples are similar and thus that sample selection biases may be small. As shown by column 1 of table 3.1, 26 percent of our sample of high-attachment workers were females, 69 percent separated from manufacturing jobs, and 61 percent had preseparation earnings exceeding $350 (1985 dollars) per week. By comparison, as shown by column 3, workers who never had positive wage or salary earnings in Pennsylvania after separating from their firms were only slightly more likely to be females or earn more than $500 per week.

This evidence about the characteristics of workers who leave our sample does alleviate one concern about our earnings loss estimates. In principle, it is possible that these workers are more able than other separators and that the reason they have no Pennsylvania earnings after they separate is that they have moved to other states where their earnings in their new firms are comparable to those in their old firms. The foregoing findings indicate that separators excluded from our sample have skills similar to workers in our sample. Whether or not these persons were more or less likely to be adversely affected by displacement is hard to say. The excluded sample contains more women, who typically have lower mobility rates following their job losses. But it also contains more workers who have high earnings. Such high-skill workers usually have higher mobility rates. Nevertheless, we believe that among these persons are workers who likely suffered greater losses than the group we study in the remainder of this monograph. For example, we find larger long-term losses when we relax our restriction requiring every person in our sample to have earnings in each calendar year to simply requiring that they have positive earnings in at least one calendar year following their separations.

Equally important as concerns about the fate of workers who leave our sample are concerns about how representative our sample is of

Table 3.1. Worker Characteristics in Pennsylvania Administrative Data, Displaced Worker Survey, and Current Population Survey Samples

Characteristic	Pennsylvania Administrative Records			Displaced Workers Survey		CPS
	All separators	Mass layoff separators	Dropout separators	All full-time respondents	High-tenure respondents	1986
	(1)	(2)	(3)	(4)	(5)	(6)
Age & gender						
Average age	41.8	41.8	43.3	–	40.5	–
Percent female	26%	23%	29%	34%	27%	40%
Preseparation industry						
Manufacturing	69%	76%	66%	48%	56%	31%
Other goods	3	4	3	13	13	8
Transportation, communications	6	5	8	8	10	8
Other services	21	15	23	32	22	52
Weekly wages (1985 dollars) prior to separation						
Less than $237	16	16	17	30	16	25
$237-$350	23	22	21	27	22	25
$351-$500	33	34	30	22	29	25
More than $500	28	29	32	21	32	25

NOTES: The table reports characteristics for the following groups of workers: (1) Pennsylvania workers with wage or salary earnings in each calendar year from 1974 through 1986, who were born between 1930 and 1959, and who had worked continuously with the same firm since at least 1974 before separating from those firms between 1980 and 1986; (2) Same as (1) except includes only workers separating from firms that had experienced large employment reductions; (3) Same as (1) except workers who never had positive Pennsylvania wage and salary earnings after their separations; (4) DWS respondents displaced from full-time jobs between 1981 and 1986; (5) DWS respondents born between 1930 and 1959, who had six or more years tenure when they were displaced between 1981 and 1986; (6) Full-time workers who responded to the January 1986 Current Population Survey. Weekly wages displaced workers nationwide. The most striking difference between our sample of separators and respondents to the DWS or the CPS is the smaller percentage of workers in our sample who were females and the larger percentage who separated from manufacturing jobs. As shown in column 4 of table 3.1, females and manufacturing workers accounted for 34 percent and 48 percent, respectively, of the 1986 DWS respondents displaced from full-time jobs. As shown in column 6, 40 percent of the January 1986 CPS respondents were females, and 31 percent were employed in manufacturing. Further, the predisplacement earnings of DWS respondents were significantly lower than either the earnings of all CPS respondents or of workers in our sample.

It is, of course, no surprise that characteristics of displaced workers differ from the workforce as a whole. Flaim and Seghal (1985) and others have reported such differences using the DWS. What is less clear is why the characteristics of workers in our sample differ from those of displaced workers in the DWS. One reason is that Pennsylvania has a greater share of large primary and fabricated metals firms than other states and that these firms experienced large employment declines during the 1980s. When we exclude workers from these firms, the percentage of workers in the resulting sample who separated from manufacturing firms declines modestly from 69 to 63 percent.

A more important reason that characteristics of displaced workers in our sample differ from the DWS is that it consists only of persons with six or more years of tenure. When we exclude persons from the DWS who report that they had fewer that 6 years of tenure when they lost their jobs or were born before 1930, we find that the characteristics of workers in the resulting DWS sample are more similar to our sample of high-attachment separators. As shown by column 5 of table 3.1, 27 percent of the high-tenure 1986 DWS respondents were females, 56 percent lost jobs from the manufacturing sector, and 61 percent earned more than $350 per week on their predisplacement job.

Another striking difference between worker characteristics in the Pennsylvania and DWS samples is the percentages of high-tenure workers displaced from other goods-producing jobs. Further analysis indicated that most of these persons were employed in the construction industry. The relatively large fraction of high-tenure displaced workers from the construction industry surprised us because that industry is typically characterized by short-term employment relationships. We have no explanation for the differences between this percentage in the two samples other than to observe that we did not find such large numbers of high-tenure displaced construction workers in our administrative data. Nonetheless, the similarity between the characteristics of high-tenure DWS respondents and our sample of separators suggests that it may be reasonable to infer that our findings reflect the experiences of high-tenure, prime-age displaced workers generally.[11]

3.4 Estimates Based on Conventional Earnings Loss Estimators

We have shown that estimates of the costs borne by dislocated workers depend on how we interpret their subsequent labor force attachment. The large size of our sample of separators, the long earnings histories, and the sample of nondisplaced workers in our administrative data also allow us to explore the sensitivity of earnings loss estimates to various assumptions about the time series patterns of worker earnings. For example, we find that our estimates of the earnings losses experienced by the sample of separators whose earnings were depicted in figures 3.1 and 3.3 depend on our interpretation of their predisplacement earnings losses and on estimates of how much their earnings would have grown had they not lost their jobs.

To underscore the potential importance of these issues when using administrative data and to motivate our development of a more formal statistical model of earnings losses in chapter 4, we analyze the 1986 annual earnings losses of the workers who separated from their firms during the first quarter of 1982. Our estimates are based on two different estimators of displaced worker earnings losses that have been employed in the displacement literature. The first estimator is simply the average difference between postdisplacement and predisplacement earnings of displaced workers. This "pre-post" estimator is similar to that often used in the DWS studies. The second estimator is the difference between age-adjusted earnings growth of displaced and nondisplaced workers. This "difference in differences" estimator, which is borrowed from the program evaluation literature,[12] has been used in some of the ILAB studies.[13] It explicitly takes into account the earnings growth that displaced workers would have experienced had they remained with their firms. In addition, besides its explicit controls for age differences, this estimator also implicitly controls for differences between workers' fixed characteristics such as their sex, race, or schooling.

To see how the "pre-post" and "difference in differences" estimators differ from each other, consider the following model of worker earnings:

$$(3.1) \quad y_{it} = \alpha_i + \gamma_t + x_{it}\beta + D_{it}\delta + \varepsilon_{it}.$$

In equation (3.1), y_{it} is worker i's earnings in period t; α_i represents worker's unmeasured fixed characteristics; γ_t represents economy-wide earnings changes; x_{it} is a quadratic in age; D_{it} equals 1 if the worker separated from his or her firm in year s and $t > s$ and equals zero otherwise; and ε_{it} is a serially uncorrelated error.[14] According to (3.1) workers' earnings may differ because their measured or unmeasured characteristics differ or because their separation statuses differ. This ambiguity is a particularly important concern in studies that estimate earnings losses by comparing postdisplacement earnings of displaced and nondisplaced workers (e.g., Seitchik and Zornitsky 1989). As (3.1) indicates, these estimates may be biased if displaced workers had unmeasured characteristics that made them more likely to have low earnings. If this is the case, the differences between postdisplacement earnings of displaced and nondisplaced workers confound the effects of displacement and the differences between their unmeasured characteristics.

We can eliminate the foregoing ambiguity by calculating the difference between current (time t) earnings and earnings in a year $(s - k)$ prior to displacement:

$$(3.2) \quad y_{it} - y_{is-k} = (\gamma_t - \gamma_{s-k}) + (x_{it} - x_{is-k})\beta + D_{it}\delta$$
$$+ (\varepsilon_{it} - \varepsilon_{is-k}).$$

In equation (3.2), earnings growth depends on economywide or sectorwide changes, age, and whether the employee had been displaced. The dependence of growth in worker earnings on these factors underscores the potential shortcoming of "pre-post" estimates. Such estimates treat the difference between post- and predisplacement earnings as having resulted from job loss. However, according to (3.2) this presumption is unlikely to be correct. Earnings of displaced workers may be changing because the economy is changing or because they are older and have more labor market experience.

The different determinants of their earnings growth underscore the value to a study of worker dislocation of a comparison group made up of nondisplaced workers. The comparison group's earnings growth identifies the coefficients for the first two terms in equation (3.2). This strategy allows displaced worker earnings histories to identify the effect of displacement. Therefore, given the equation (3.1) earnings model, the difference between earnings growth (adjusted for age) of displaced workers and the comparison group is an unbiased estimate of the costs of worker dislocation.

These points are made more concretely in table 3.2, where we present alternative estimates of the earnings losses incurred by workers who separated from their firms during the first quarter of 1982. This set of estimates also indicates how loss estimates depend on post-separation attachment to the wage and salary workforce. Indeed, as shown by Panel A of table 3.2, "pre-post" estimates of workers' earnings losses depend to a substantial degree on their subsequent labor force attachment. Earnings of displaced workers were $9,191 lower in 1986 than in 1981, one year prior to their separations. When we limit our sample of separators to workers with wage or salary earnings during 1986, the earnings drop falls to $3,389. Finally, when we limit our sample of separators to displaced workers with wage or salary earnings in every calendar year—about one-half of the displaced—the annual earnings loss falls to only $2,483. Thus, when we focus only on workers who remain highly attached to the Pennsylvania wage and salary workforce, the estimated earnings losses are only one-fourth as large as the apparent losses for the full sample of separators.

Turning to the comparison group-based estimates in the last column of Panel B, we find that they are larger than the corresponding "pre-post" estimates. These larger loss estimates reflect the earnings growth experienced by similarly aged workers who remained employed at their firms. As shown by the last row in Panel B of table

3.2, the "difference in differences" estimate of the high-attachment sample's annual earnings losses is $5,030 compared with the "pre-post" estimate of only $2,483. The simple "pre-post" estimates understate the costs of worker dislocation because the comparison group's earnings grew modestly between 1981 and 1986. That earnings growth suggests that had displaced workers remained with their old employers their earnings also would have grown substantially.

The other columns in table 3.2 indicate that even the "difference in differences" estimates may be misleading. One problem is that the estimates vary depending on the predisplacement year, $s - k$. As shown in the last row of the table, the estimated earnings losses for the sample of separators who remained attached to Pennsylvania's wage and salary workforce range from $5,030 when using 1981 as the predisplacement base year to $6,528 when using 1980 as the predisplacement base year. Although this variability may not be surprising given the standard errors associated with the estimates, the main reason that our estimates vary depending on which year we use as the predisplacement year is that displaced worker earnings grow more slowly or even decline in the years prior to displacement. This pattern is seen more clearly in the behavior of the "pre-post" estimates in Panel A. For example, the 1986 earnings of high-attachment separators are $4,287 below their 1979 levels, but only $2,483 below their 1981 levels. This decline could result because the events that lead to worker separations cause their earnings to grow more slowly or even decline before their displacements.

We also can observe the foregoing problem with the "difference in differences" estimates in figure 3.3. The figure shows that the earnings of separators actually began to diverge from those of the stayers several quarters before they left their firms. One explanation for that divergence is that firms initially respond to adverse economic conditions by reducing employee hours, temporarily laying off segments of their workforce, and cutting real wages. That explanation suggests that displaced workers experience earnings losses prior to their job losses as a result of the same forces that ultimately lead to their separations. In this sense, the preseparation earnings declines are a part of the displacement effect that we are trying to measure.

An alternative explanation for the divergence between the earnings patterns of separators and nondisplaced workers suggests that the "difference in differences" estimates in the last row of table 3.2 are biased no matter which preseparation year we use. This explanation is based on the evidence in column 3 of Panel B, which shows that between 1974 and 1979, age-adjusted earnings of separators usually grew more slowly than those of nondisplaced workers. For example, the earnings of separators who remained attached to the Pennsylvania wage or salary workforce grew by $1,517 less than the earnings of those who stayed with their firms through 1986. Therefore, simple "difference in differences" estimates are likely to be biased if employers select for displacement those employees with more slowly growing or even declining productivity. This second explanation implies that some of the postdisplacement earnings gap between separators and nondisplaced workers would have existed even if these employees had not been displaced and their firms had not experienced economic difficulties.

The reason we require a more complex estimator than our simple "difference in differences" estimator is that our long earnings histories make clear that worker earnings are inconsistent with the model described in equation (3.1). If earnings are generated as in (3.1), earnings growth (adjusted for age) should be the same for the separators and nondisplaced workers in the years prior to displacement. This specification does not allow for differences between predisplacement earnings growth of displaced and nondisplaced workers to depend on anything other than differences in their ages. But, during the predisplacement period, we find that age-adjusted earnings of separators grew more slowly than those of their nondisplaced counterparts.

Accordingly, this evidence suggests that worker earnings are better summarized by an alternative model. In this formulation, earnings also depend on an individual-specific deterministic trend, $\omega_i t$. Equation (3.1) now becomes:

$$(3.3) \qquad y_{it} = \alpha_i + \omega_i t + \gamma_t + x_{it}\beta + D_{it}\delta + \varepsilon_{it}.$$

After differencing (3.3) using predisplacement earnings, y_{is-k}, the potential bias associated with the "difference in differences" estimator becomes clear:

$$(3.4) \qquad y_{it} - y_{is-k} = \omega_i(t - (s-k)) + (\gamma_t - \gamma_{s-k})$$
$$+ (x_{it} - x_{is-k}))\beta + D_{it}\delta + (\varepsilon_{it} - \varepsilon_{is-k}).$$

Table 3.2 1986 Earnings Losses for Nonagricultural Workers Displaced in 1982:I

	Number of observations	1979 earnings	1979-1974	1986-1978	1986-1979	1986-1980	1986-1981
Panel A: Differences Between Pre- and Postdisplacement Earnings							
All displaced workers	425	$22,862 (492)	$2,154 (328)	$-11,873 (668)	$-12,020 (659)	$-10,934 (638)	$-9,191 (632)
Displaced workers with 1986 earnings	260	23,412 (635)	1,931 (446)	-5,450 (733)	-5,690 (722)	-4,967 (717)	-3,389 (703)
Displaced workers with 1974-1986 earnings	188	24,927 (698)	1,825 (573)	-4,145 (773)	-4,287 (786)	-4,094 (795)	-2,483 (745)
Panel B: Differences Between Displaced Workers' and Stayers' Earnings Growth							
All displaced workers			$-980 (330)	$-13,287 (472)	$-13,376 (468)	$-13,242 (448)	$-11,591 (428)
Displaced workers with 1986 earnings			-1,232 (421)	-6,883 (594)	-7,061 (589)	-7,301 (564)	-5,818 (537)
Displaced workers with 1974-1986 earnings			-1,517 (521)	-5,594 (732)	-5,675 (726)	-6,528 (696)	-5,030 (662)

NOTE: Estimates based on a 5 percent sample of all Pennsylvania nonmanufacturing employees with eight or more years of tenure in their firm when displaced in 1982. In Panel B, the estimates control for a quadratic in age. The stayers sample includes 8,232 manufacturing employees with eight or more years of tenure in 1982 who stayed with their firms through 1986. Average earnings for stayers in 1979 was $26,284. Standard errors are in parentheses.

The earnings growth of those employees who stayed with their firms cannot identify both differences in individual, ω_i, and aggregate, $\gamma_t - \gamma_{s-k}$, earnings growth. Therefore, earnings growth differences between separators and stayers partly reflects differences that would have existed even if no separation had occurred. One way to account for individual earnings growth differences is to use the differences between displaced and nondisplaced worker earnings growth from 1974-1979 to estimate what the differences in their earnings growth would have been between 1979 and 1986 had there been no separations from their firms. Such "second difference in differences" estimates are approximately 20 percent lower than the estimates shown in Panel B.

3.5 Conclusion

This chapter examined how state administrative records could be used in studies of worker dislocation. Such records have long earnings histories free from the response biases that may arise in interview data. Moreover, we have shown that valuable information about job changes is available from administrative records, but must be constructed with considerable care. In addition, studies that use such data must confront the problems that these records do not explicitly distinguish between quits and layoffs and do not record the earnings of persons who have left the state. In this chapter we argued that for samples of high-tenure workers these problems are likely to be less important.

Our preliminary analysis of a subsample of separators indicated that when high-tenure workers separate from their firms, they experience substantial earnings reductions. In the long term, these earnings losses may amount to approximately $4,000 to $5,000 per year, or between 20 and 25 percent below what average earnings would have been in the absence of displacement. However, because our administrative data provide long earnings histories, we are able to identify several difficulties associated with this finding. When developing our formal statistical model of displaced worker earnings losses in chapter 4, we take these difficulties explicitly into account. Our empirical analyses in chapters 5 and 6 indicate that how we treat these issues has a substantial effect on the magnitude of displaced workers' long-term earnings losses.

NOTES

1. See *Employment and Earnings*, U.S. Department of Labor, various issues; and Jacobson (1988).

2. Employers report their employees total earnings. Unlike Social Security earnings data, these data are not top coded. For our own data processing convenience, we have top coded earnings over $100,000 per quarter. We also obtained information on the workers' receipt of unemployment insurance benefits and TAA payments by quarter.

3. The sample is based on the last two digits of workers' Social Security numbers.

4. The reports actually identify employment levels of individual establishments. However, the coding schemes vary from year to year and we thus have not been able to make use of data on employment trends of workers' establishments.

5. Although we have less demographic information on workers than we would like, we are fortunate to have as much as we do. Pennsylvania was one of the few states to obtain demographic information from the Social Security Administration before concern for privacy caused them to stop supplying such information on individuals.

6. Unless stated otherwise, all dollar figures in this monograph have been deflated by the Consumer Price Index and are given in 1987 dollars.

7. Both the displaced and nondisplaced workers had eight or more years of service with their firms as of the first quarter of 1982.

8. In figure 3.2, the upward spike in the employment rate at the quarter of separation is a consequence of the way separations are dated; all workers had to have positive earnings in their quarters of separation—otherwise we would have dated their separations one quarter earlier.

9. In the future we hope to obtain data indicating whether workers have positive earnings anywhere in the United States. This information would provide a better picture of the labor market activity of workers with zero reported earnings.

10. Some workers are also excluded if they were unemployed for more than one year following their displacements. An example of such workers are those displaced during the fourth quarter, who have no earnings during the entire subsequent year. However, some workers unemployed for more than one and one-half years following their job losses would be included in the sample if they were displaced during the first or second quarter and did not find a job until the third or fourth quarter of the following year.

11. Interestingly, because Pennsylvania workers are paid only modestly more than all U.S. workers, differences in local wages probably do not explain the pay differences observed in table 3.1. In 1980, production and supervisory workers in manufacturing earned $384 (1985 dollars) per week in Pennsylvania compared with $376 (1985 dollars) per week in the U.S. (see *Employment, Hours, and Earnings, States and Area, 1939-82* Volume II: New Hampshire-Wyoming. U.S. Department of Labor, Bulletin 1370-17, p. 710, January 1984; 1991 *Economic Report of the President,* tables B-44, B-58, pp. 336, 351). We converted 1980 dollars to 1985 dollars by multiplying the 1980 figures by 1.306.

12. For examples of these models see Ashenfelter (1978), Bassi (1984), Ashenfelter and Card (1985), Heckman and Robb (1985), LaLonde (1986), Card and Sullivan (1988).

13. Ruhm (1991a) employs a similar technique.

14. Model (3.1) implies that any earnings losses after separation are permanent. Because we are comparing only one postdisplacement year, 1986, to several predisplacement years, 1978 to 1981, that assumption has no impact on the results in table 3.1. We relax this assumption in chapter 4 when we consider models that allow the displacement effects to vary over time.

4
Econometric Issues
in the Estimation
of Earnings Losses

In chapter 3, we examined the earnings histories of experienced workers who were displaced in the first quarter of 1982 and similar workers who remained with their firms through the end of 1986. We noted that the significant differences between the earnings histories of those two groups strongly suggested that displacement led to large losses in earnings. We also noted a number of issues likely to affect estimates of those losses. In this chapter we discuss these issues more fully and present our strategy for summarizing the evidence on the magnitude of displaced worker earnings losses. We begin by specifying more precisely the definition of earnings loss used in this monograph. Next we present our basic estimation strategy. This is followed by a discussion of possible statistical biases that might, under certain circumstances, affect our estimates. Finally, we show how the basic estimation strategy can be extended to allow estimates to depend on various characteristics of workers and their firms.

4.1 The Meaning of Earnings Losses Due to Displacement

Figure 4.1 summarizes the qualitative characteristics of displaced and nondisplaced worker earnings histories. As suggested in chapter 3, earnings of displaced workers rise until two to three years prior to their separations from their firms. Then, during the years immediately prior to their separations (D-C in figure 4.1), their earnings begin to decline. When they actually lose their jobs, their earnings fall sharply (C in figure 4.1). Finally, their earnings recover at a modest rate during the years following their separations. In contrast, the earnings of similar workers who were not displaced continue to grow over the entire time period (D-B in figure 4.1)—suggesting that had displaced workers not lost their jobs, their earnings also would have grown.

Figure 4.1 Stylized Earnings Histories of Displaced Worker and Similar Nondisplaced Worker

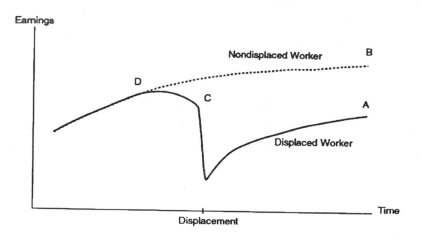

The stylized earnings histories depicted in figure 4.1 can be used to illustrate several possible definitions of the earnings loss due to displacement. One definition is the simple difference between postdisplacement earnings and earnings immediately prior to displacement (A-C in figure 4.1). A second possibility is the difference between postdisplacement earnings and earnings several years prior to displacement (A-D in figure 4.1). A third possibility is the difference between postdisplacement earnings and the earnings workers would have received had they not been displaced (A-B in figure 4.1). The latter amount depends on the earnings of nondisplaced workers in a comparison group. That group might include nondisplaced workers who had similar earnings histories and characteristics to the displaced workers before the events that led to their displacement began. Our analysis of 1982 separators in chapter 3 indicated that these definitions yielded substantially different estimates of earnings losses. Thus, the estimated magnitude of displaced worker earnings losses clearly turns on the rationale for adopting one definition over the others.

As noted in chapter 2, much of the previous dislocation literature adopted (often implicitly) the first earnings loss definition. Studies using the DWS had little choice but to employ this simple "pre-post" definition because the DWS does not include a comparison group of nondisplaced workers and even for displaced workers includes information only on earnings immediately prior to displacement. However, earnings declines that occur prior to worker separations are just as injurious as declines that occur after they actually leave their employer. Similarly, the loss of earnings growth that they would otherwise have expected is just as significant in any welfare calculation as an actual drop in earnings. Accordingly, for the purposes of understanding the link between a firm's success and the well-being of its employees or for determining the amount of compensation necessary to make adversely affected workers indifferent to policy changes, the third definition is the most meaningful.

Simply put, we wish to compare the typical displaced worker's actual earnings with what they would have been in the hypothetical case in which the worker was not displaced. This definition of the loss is not, however, sufficiently precise. In particular, it does not fully specify the meaning of "not being displaced." One possibility would be to compare actual earnings with those that could have expected had the worker not been displaced at the particular date of separation. If we let y_{it} denote the earnings of worker i at date t and let $D_{is} = 1$ if worker i was displaced at date s (and $D_{is} = 0$ otherwise) then this definition of the loss would lead us to estimate the quantity

$$(4.1) \qquad E(y_{it} \mid D_{is} = 1) - E(y_{it} \mid D_{is} = 0).$$

This definition does not rule out the possibility that worker i was displaced at some time other than date s. Instead of this definition, however, we prefer a stronger definition of not being displaced. Not only do we require nondisplaced workers to remain at their firms at date s, but at all other dates in our sampling frame. Therefore, we attempt to estimate the quantity

$$(4.2) \qquad E(y_{i\tau} \mid D_{is} = 1) - E(y_{it} \mid D_{iv} = 0 \text{ for all } v).$$

Because the alternative to displacement in (4.2) rules out displacement at any time in the future in addition to displacement at date s, the losses calculated this way should be larger than those implied by (4.1).[1]

Relative to the definition in equation (4.1), the quantity in equation (4.2) is a cleaner measure of the importance of job loss to a worker's career. In particular, measure (4.1) partially depends on how workers who are displaced at a given date fare relative to workers displaced shortly before or after that date. Such a comparison is not likely to be the one that most interests policymakers. An additional advantage of (4.2) over (4.1) is that it compares job losers at different dates to a common standard. This simplifies the interpretation of several of our results. Finally, the quantity (4.1) can be calculated from (4.2) if we have additional information on how $\text{Prob}(D_{iv} = 1 | D_{is} = 0)$ varies with v and s. Thus obtaining estimates of (4.2) can be viewed as a useful preliminary step in the estimation of (4.1).[2]

Even specification (4.2) is insufficiently precise to describe the problem we are attempting to address. Besides whether a worker was displaced, the magnitudes of both expectations in (4.2) depend on the additional information on which we condition. We can write (4.2) more precisely if, in addition to displacement status, we condition on the information set, I_i,

$$(4.3) \qquad E(y_{it} \mid D_{is} = 1, I_i) - E(y_{it} \mid D_{iv} = 0 \text{ for all } v, I_i).$$

The information set I_i in equation (4.3) includes worker characteristics, but it also has a temporal dimension that potentially has an important effect on our earnings loss definitions. To see how this effect arises let I_{it} denote information about worker i that is available at time t. One possible definition of earnings losses would set I_i in equation (4.3) equal to I_{is}.

$$(4.4) \qquad E(y_{it} \mid D_{is} = 1, I_{is}) - E(y_{it} \mid D_{iv} = 0 \text{ for all } v, I_{is}).$$

In equation (4.4), the expected loss at time t depends on the information available at the time of separation. Thus (4.4) denotes the change in earnings expectation that occurs at the time workers are displaced.

Our view, however, is that the earnings loss definition given in equation (4.4) captures only part of the adverse effects associated with displacement. By the time the reduction in force actually occurs, the declining firm's fortunes may have been at least partially evident for some time. Indeed, we have already seen in chapter 3 that the earnings of displaced workers begin to decline around three years prior to their separations. Therefore, it seems very likely that their expected future earnings would also have begun to decline. In general, if the forces of structural change work over a significant period of time so that the firm's fortunes are continually eroding, workers' expected earnings may have largely absorbed the effects of that structural change by the time they leave their firms. In that case, employee separations might not reveal much additional information about their future earnings prospects, and as a result the loss corresponding to equation (4.4) would be relatively small.

Because earnings may absorb the adverse effects of structural change prior to worker displacements, it is important to estimate expected earnings prior to these changes. Therefore, we choose to focus on the more comprehensive definition of earnings losses that compares earnings of displaced workers to the earnings that they expected to receive at some date p periods prior to their separations. More formally, we estimate

$$(4.5) \qquad E(y_{it} \mid D_{is} = 1, I_{is\text{-}p}) - E(y_{it} \mid D_{iv} = 0 \text{ for all } v, I_{is\text{-}p}),$$

where p is sufficiently large that the events that eventually lead to displacement have not begun at time $s - p$. The quantity (4.5) is the change in expected earnings, if, at time $s - p$, it was revealed that the worker would be displaced at date s rather than being able to keep his or her job indefinitely. When structural changes take a significant amount of time to unfold, it is necessary that $s - p$ precede those changes in order to capture displacement's full effects on earnings.

Before we can implement the foregoing definition we need to specify the variables in the information set $I_{is\text{-}p}$. These variables should be determinants of earnings whether or not workers are displaced. We clearly want to control as best we can for the standard demographic variables that influence earnings.[3] Our data allow us to go even further, because they allow us to condition on the industries and even on the firms that displaced workers were attached to before they lost their jobs.[4] However, the problem with such controls is that even workers who are fortunate enough to retain their jobs with firms that layoff other workers may experience some earnings losses. An expression like

(4.6) $E(y_{it} \mid D_{is} = 1, i$ employed by firm f at $s - p)$

$- E(y_{it} \mid D_{iv} = 0$ for all v, i employed by firm f at $s - p)$,

does not capture the full impact of the events that led to displacement, because it captures only the effects specifically associated with job loss.

Our preferred definition of displaced worker earnings losses limits I_{is-p} to general characteristics of a worker and his or her firm that are known at date $s - p$ to affect earnings. This definition does not mean that no firm characteristics should be included in the set of variables that determine expected earnings. For instance, suppose it is widely known that workers in larger firms have earnings that rise more rapidly than those in smaller firms. In that case, it is appropriate to base conditional earnings forecasts on the size of the firm that the worker was employed in at date $s - p$. We argue, however, that expected earnings, in the event that workers are able to keep their jobs, should not be lowered by the knowledge that workers similar to themselves are going to be laid off.

We do not believe that policymakers concerned with the ramifications of potential policy interventions in areas such as international trade and environmental protection would be comforted to learn that workers who would lose their jobs would suffer no greater earnings losses than the workers who remained with the affected firms if, in fact, the earnings of both groups would be devastated. Likewise, in attempting to understand the importance of workers' attachment to particular firms, we need to see variation in outcomes of similar workers in different firms. Thus our preferred definition of the earnings loss due to displacement is that given by equation (4.5) where I_{is-p} is limited to characteristics of a worker and his or her firm that would, at date $s - p$, be thought to affect earnings.

In order to make clear the empirical importance of including or excluding firm controls, we report estimates based on both measures in chapters 5 and 6. We do so for two reasons. First, we believe the difference between equations (4.5) and (4.6) sheds some light on the interpretation of the estimated earnings losses. Second, that difference can serve as an indirect indicator of the losses imposed by structural change on workers who retain their jobs.[5]

4.2 Basic Statistical Model

In addition to the problem of defining earnings losses, we also have the statistical problem of estimating those losses. To estimate these losses we specify a statistical model that exploits the principal strengths of our data—its large sample size and its long time span—to obtain a very detailed picture of the pattern of earnings losses both across time and across workers. We identify the displacement effect with a subset of the model's parameters that captures the varied effects that this event can have on earnings histories. In our specification, the effect of displacement on earnings depends on the length of time since the separation date. For instance, immediately after displacement, unemployment is likely to be a significant source of earnings losses. But, in the long run, less earnings losses are more likely to depend on the amount of specific human capital possessed by workers before their displacements and the rate at which they accumulate new capital after displacement.

Understanding the temporal pattern of earnings losses is important for at least two reasons. First, the aggregate loss borne by displaced workers depends on the effect of displacement on their earnings for the entire rest of their careers. Because we are able to follow the temporal pattern of earnings losses for over six years after displacement, we can reasonably assess the speed with which earnings recover and thus estimate the cumulative loss associated with displacement. Second, the potential for various policy measures to compensate workers for job loss occasioned by freer trade or tighter environmental protection depends critically on when they incur these losses. If displacement reduces earnings for a relatively short period following separation as a result of unemployment, then programs that provide supplemental unemployment benefits may adequately compensate displaced workers. If, however, the drop in earnings is long term, persisting even after workers find stable employment, then such programs alone will not be enough.

Besides the temporal pattern being important, there is also ample reason to believe that earnings losses depend on characteristics of the affected workers such as their sex, age, or former firm's industry. For instance, the various factors discussed in chapter 1 that may lead to earnings premia for workers are likely to be more important in some industries than others. Similarly, a displaced worker's ability and inclination to make new investments in human capital likely depend on age and possibly on sex. An understanding of the dependence of earnings losses on worker characteristics would be valuable to policymakers for at least two reasons. First, those concerned with the consequences of a policy intervention that adversely affects a particular group would want to know the probable size of the losses that would be suffered by that specific group rather than by the average worker. Second, if the time pattern of losses is known to differ across groups of workers in a specific manner, it may be possible to tailor different compensation schemes to different groups of affected workers.

Unfortunately, our twin goals of allowing for a flexible pattern of loss estimates over time and for dependence of estimates on worker characteristics conflict to a certain extent. For instance, the estimates underlying figure 3.3 in chapter 3 are relatively successful in displaying the intertemporal pattern of earnings losses. However, they do not show how losses vary across groups of workers. Simply splitting the sample of experienced workers who underlie those estimates (those displaced in the first quarter of 1982) into subgroups of workers defined by characteristics such as age, sex, and industry is not feasible. Even with the large data set that we are employing, the resulting subgroups would be too small to produce statistically reliable estimates.

In order to allow for variation of the estimates across both time and worker characteristics, it is necessary to pool information from various cohorts of displaced workers. A convenient way to do this is to introduce a set of dummy variables, each of which is one a particular number of quarters before or after a worker is displaced and zero otherwise. In particular, let $D_{it}^k = 1$ if, in period t, worker i had been displaced k quarters earlier.[6] Alternatively, $D_{it}^k = 1$ if worker i was displaced in quarter $t - k$. By restricting attention to these dummy variables, we formalize the idea that, for example, a worker displaced in 1982 was in much the same position in 1985 as a worker displaced in 1981 was in 1984.

The basic statistical specification on which we base the estimates presented below assumes that a worker's earnings at a given date depend on displacement through the above set of dummy variables and on some additional controls:

$$(4.7) \qquad y_{it} = \alpha_i + \gamma_t + x_{it}\beta + \sum_{k \geq -m} D_{it}^k \delta_k + \varepsilon_{it}.$$

The complete set of dummy variables, D_{it}^k $k = -m, -(m-1), \ldots, 0, 1, 2, \ldots$ represents the event of displacement. In particular, δk is the effect of displacement on a worker's earnings k quarters following its occurrence, or if k is negative, $|k|$ quarters prior to job loss. The remainder of the variables in (4.7) were included in an attempt to control for other general factors that influence earnings. The vector x_{it} consists of observed, time-varying characteristics of the worker. In this study, these are limited to age, age squared, sex, and interactions of these variables. The γ_t's, which are the coefficients on a set of dummy variables for each quarter in the sample period, capture the general time pattern of earnings in the economy. Specification (4.7) also allows for the existence of permanent differences across workers in observed and unobserved characteristics. The impact of such fixed factors is summarized for each worker by the coefficient α_i. For example, more highly educated or more highly motivated workers who consistently earn more than other workers have high values of α_i. In particular, it is important to note that, given the presence in (4.7) of the worker-specific fixed effect, α_i, additional information on characteristics such as completed years of education that do not change over time are of no value; the effects of such variables are completely summarized by the fixed effects. Finally, the error term, ε_{it}, in specification (4.7) is assumed to be of constant variance and to be uncorrelated across individuals and time.

The specification discussed in chapter 3 is a special case of (4.7) where $\delta_k = 0$ for all $k < 0$ and $\delta_k = \delta$ for all $k \geq 0$. Specification (4.7) allows displacement's effects on earnings to be felt up to m quarters prior to separation and for those effects to quickly disappear or, alternatively, to persist indefinitely. By freeing up the specification to allow the effects of displacement to vary over time, we achieve one of the goals set out above—that of allowing in a flexible way for a complex temporal pattern of loss and recovery. In section 4.4 we discuss how our second goal—allowing for flexibility across workers—can be achieved, but first we consider some issues relating to the specification that can be more clearly appreciated without those additional complications.

As noted above, expression (4.5) is our preferred definition of the earnings loss due to displacement. It compares the expected earnings at time t of an individual who was displaced at time s with those of a worker who was never displaced. In terms of our statistical model equation (4.7), at time t, a worker who is displaced at time s has $D_{it}^{t-s} = 1$ and all other displacement dummies equal to zero. In contrast, a worker who is never displaced will have all of the displacement dummies equal to zero. Thus the two terms making up the quantity (4.5) can be expressed as

$$(4.8) \quad E(y_{it} \mid D_{is} = 1, I_{is\text{-}p}) = \delta_{t\text{-}s} + E(\alpha_i + \gamma_t + x_{it}\beta + \varepsilon_{it} \mid D_{is} = 1, I_{is\text{-}p})$$

and

$$(4.9) \quad E(y_{it} \mid D_{iv} = 0 \text{ for all } v, I_{is\text{-}p}) = E(\alpha_i + \gamma_t + x_{it}\beta + \varepsilon_{it} \mid D_{iv} = 0 \text{ for all } v, I_{is\text{-}p}).$$

As we noted in section 4.1, the most appropriate information set, $I_{is\text{-}p}$, includes general characteristics of the worker known at time $s - p$ to be determinants of present and future earnings. In terms of the variables included in specification (4.7), these include α_i and x_{it} which are, respectively, permanent characteristics of a worker and time-varying variables whose path would be known at time $s - p$. Thus, $E(\alpha_i \mid D_{is} = 1, I_{is\text{-}p}) = E(\alpha_i \mid D_{iv} = 0 \text{ for all } v, I_{is\text{-}p}) = \alpha_i$ and similarly $E(x_{it}\beta \mid D_{is} = 1, I_{is\text{-}p}) = E(x_{it}\beta \mid D_{iv} = 0$ for all v, $I_{is\text{-}p}) = x_{it}\beta$. The realization of γ_t will not be known at time $s - p$. But, we argued above that when assessing the effects of displacement, it was inappropriate to include variables in $I_{is\text{-}p}$ that, when combined with information on whether a particular worker was displaced, would provide information about the earnings of other workers. Thus, for the appropriate information set, $E(\gamma_t \mid D_{is} = 1, I_{is\text{-}p}) = E(\gamma_t \mid D_{iv} = 0$ for all v, $I_{is\text{-}p})$. This last fact, combined with our assumption about the error term in model (4.7), implies that the desired quantity, (4.5), reduces to $\delta_{t\text{-}s}$, the coefficient on the dummy variable for being t-s quarters after displacement.

Given our assumption that the error term in (4.7) is of constant variance and independent across observations, and given our unwillingness to assume, for instance, that α_i is uncorrelated with the D_{it}^k, the most efficient way to estimate equation (4.7) is by ordinary least squares with the α_i treated as the coefficients of dummy variables for the corresponding individual.[7] As is widely known, this estimator can be calculated in a computationally tractable manner, by first "sweeping out" the individual specific dummy variables, that is, by replacing all other variables with their deviations from worker-specific means. If we denote the mean of worker i's earnings by $\bar{y}_i$ and similarly for other variables, then

(4.10) $$\bar{y}_i = \alpha_i + \bar{\gamma} + \bar{x}_i\beta + \sum_{k \geq -m} \bar{D}_i^k \delta_k + \bar{\varepsilon}_i$$

and

(4.11) $$y_{it} - \bar{y}_i = \gamma_t' + (x_{it} - \bar{x}_i)\beta + \sum_{k \geq -m} (D_{it}^k - \bar{D}_i^k)\delta_k + (\varepsilon_{it} - \bar{\varepsilon}_i) \ .$$

Least squares applied to (4.11) yields the same estimates of its parameters as least squares applied to (4.7) but is computationally tractable because the α_i's have been eliminated.

Even estimation of (4.11) can be somewhat burdensome since there are a relatively large number of both the γ_t's (52, or one for each quarter) and δ_k's (48, or one for each number of quarters relative to displacement between 20 quarters before displacement and 27 quarters after displacement) and the sample size is large (roughly 1,500,000 worker-quarter observations). The computations can, however, be reduced somewhat more by computing the estimates in two steps. Specifically, for the subsample of workers who are never displaced, (4.7) reduces to

$$(4.12) \quad y_{it} = \alpha_i + \gamma_t + x_{it}\beta + \varepsilon_{it}.$$

Consistent estimates of β and the γ_t's can be obtained by estimating (4.12) using only the data on the workers who were never displaced. Denote these estimates by $\tilde{\beta}$ and $\tilde{\gamma}_t$. Then $\tilde{y}_{it} = y_{it} - \tilde{\gamma}_t - x_{it}\tilde{\beta}$ is a consistent estimate of $\alpha_i + \sum D_{it}^k \delta_k + \varepsilon_{it}$ for displaced workers. Thus we can consistently estimate the parameters of primary interest, the δ_k's, by applying least squares to

$$(4.13) \quad \tilde{y}_{it} = \alpha_i + \sum_{k \geq -m} D_{it}^k \delta_k + \varepsilon_{it}.$$

Relative to those obtained by least squares estimation of (4.11), estimates obtained from (4.13)[8] are less efficient and the estimated standard errors produced by standard software are probably optimistic in that they do not take account of the fact that $\tilde{\beta}$ and the $\tilde{\gamma}_t$'s are only estimates. However, we have found the estimates and their standard errors produced using (4.13) to be extremely close to those derived from (4.11).[9]

Implicit in our discussion of the estimation (4.7) is that it is estimable. However, it is clear that (4.7) will not be identified unless we have data on at least some displaced workers more than m quarters prior to their displacement. In particular, if we did not have such data then it would not be possible to distinguish the case in which all displaced workers have low values of the fixed effect, α_i, from the case in which the δ_k's are all negative and large in absolute value. More formally, if there were no data on displaced workers more than m quarters prior to their displacement, then for these workers, exactly one of the D_{it}^k would always be equal to 1 in each period. Thus if we had one set of least squares parameters we could always get another set, implying identical fitted values, by adding any constant to all the α_i's corresponding to displaced workers and subtracting the same constant from all of the δ_k's.[10] In this case we would only be able to estimate differences between δ_k's. That is, we could determine, for example, whether a worker suffers a greater drop in earnings 5 quarters after displacement or 10 quarters after displacement, but we would not be able to determine the absolute magnitude of either of these quantities since we would lack data on a period where we could assume there had been no effects due to displacement.

As we noted above, we have chosen to let m be 20 quarters or 5 years. This presents us with no problems of identification. Even for our first cohort of displaced workers, those who separated from their firms in the first quarter of 1980, we have 6 years of predisplacement data. We have also estimated versions of (4.7) with m set equal to values of up to 10 years. In no case did we see evidence of an effect of displacement prior to three or four years before the actual separation. Thus we feel confident in imposing the assumption that there are no displacement effects prior to 5 years before separation.[11]

4.3 Potential Biases

This monograph assesses the impact on earnings of a particular class of events that are beyond workers' control—those that affect their entire firm and cause them to lose their jobs. Accordingly, we have identified the losses due to displacement with events that happen to a worker's firm rather than directly to the worker. The fundamental source of bias in the estimation of displacement effects is thus confusion of the effects of worker-specific events with firmwide events that lead to displacement. For example, biased estimates may arise when worker-specific events or characteristics cause some workers both to be more likely to be (or appear to be) displaced and to have lower earnings independently of whether they are displaced.

One simple, but important, special case where characteristics of individuals might be associated with both displacement and direct effects on earnings arises when the characteristics in question are permanent but unobserved attributes of the workers. Such attributes, which might include years of schooling, innate intelligence, strength, motivation, and a host of other factors, partially determine an individual's level of regular earnings and quite possibly also influence the probability that the individual will be displaced. Indeed, if we were to simply compare the mean earnings of a group of displaced workers a certain period of time after their separations with those of workers who were not displaced, the difference in earnings would confound the effects of displacement with the differences in unobserved regular earnings levels, thereby yielding overestimates of the effects of displacement.[12]

It is important to note that the estimators employed below would not be biased in the situation just described. Indeed, one of the principal goals of our modeling and estimation strategy is eliminating this source of bias. In particular, the possibility of heterogeneity in permanent worker characteristics is allowed for by the inclusion of the fixed effects (the α_i's). According to model (4.7), the simple difference between the mean earnings of displaced workers k periods after displacement and the mean earnings of a randomly selected group of nondisplaced workers would have expectation equal to $\delta_k + \overline{D} - \overline{ND}$ where $\overline{D}$ and $\overline{ND}$ are the means of the α_i's for the displaced and nondisplaced workers respectively.[13] If workers with low α_i's are more likely to be displaced, $\overline{D} < \overline{ND}$. Thus the difference in mean earnings would be greater in absolute value than the true displacement effect, δ_k. Intuitively, our estimates based on model (4.7) eliminate this bias by relying only on temporal variation in earnings. That variation does not depend on the level of the fixed effect.[14] As is clear from equation (4.11), in which the fixed effects do not appear, the distribution of the α_i's is completely irrelevant to the properties of our estimator.

Other forms of correlation of individual characteristics with displacement *can* lead to biases in the estimators that we employ. For instance, when there is diversity not only in individual workers' level of regular earnings but also in their trend rates of earnings growth, and when those individual growth rates are related to the probability of displacement, our estimates of δ_k will be biased. Such a case may arise when workers with lower than average rates of earnings growth are more likely to be displaced than those with higher rates of growth. In this case our estimation technique will overstate the effects of displacement.

This issue can be analyzed in the context of the following extension of model (4.7):

$$(4.14) \quad y_{it} = \alpha_i + \omega_i t + \gamma_t + x_{it}\beta + \sum_{k \geq -m} D_{it}^k \delta_k + \varepsilon_{it}.$$

Model (4.14) differs from (4.7) in its inclusion of a set of worker-specific time trends, $\omega_i t$. As we noted above, estimating (4.7) is equivalent to estimating (4.11). Thus, if (4.14) is the correct model, our estimates will be based on

$$(4.15) \quad y_{it} - \bar{y}_i = \gamma'_t + (x_{it} - \bar{x}_i)\beta \sum_{k \geq -m} (D_{it}^k - \bar{D}_i^k)\delta_k$$
$$+ \bar{\omega}_i(t - \bar{t}) + (\varepsilon_{it} - \bar{\varepsilon}_i)$$

where the quantity $\bar{\omega}_i(t - \bar{t}) + (\varepsilon_{it} - \bar{\varepsilon}_i)$ can be thought of as a composite error term for the model. If displaced workers tend to have lower values of ω_i, then this error term would be negatively correlated with the variables $D_{it}^k - \bar{D}_i^k$, which would impart a negative bias to the estimates of the δ_k's.[15]

It is possible to eliminate the potential bias just discussed by computing least squares estimates of model (4.14). Computationally, this would amount to estimating a regression model similar to (4.11) in which all the variables were measured as deviations from a worker-specific time trend rather than simply from a worker-specific mean.[16] In other work, we have computed such estimates and found them to differ little from those based on the simpler fixed effects specification.[17] Our estimates of the effects of displacement on earnings several years prior to separation show why this should be the case. As we noted above, these estimates tend to be approximately zero four or more years prior to separation. However, it is clear from (4.15) that any bias imparted by heterogeneity in the ω_i's will affect all of the δ_k's, including those measuring the effects of displacement several years prior to separation. The fact that we do not see displacement effects more than three years prior to separation shows that heterogeneity in worker-specific trends is not an important source of bias in the results we present below.

The previous paragraph points up another advantage of the long time series provided by the Pennsylvania data. Because we have data on workers' earnings long before their separations, we can estimate the effects of displacement on their earnings well before separation occurs. These estimates can be used as a form of specification test. If a proposed model were misspecified, it is likely that this misspecification would cause all of the estimated displacement effects, including those more than three years prior to separation, to be nonzero and thus lead us to reject the specification. This point is expanded upon below in the discussion of the empirical results.

Another form of misspecification that may lead to biased estimates arises when firms select for displacement employees whose performance was unusually poor in the periods immediately prior to separation. In this case workers may be selected for displacement partly on the basis of the realized value of the error term in our model of earnings. To analyze this issue it is convenient to assume that in addition to the error term, ε_{it}, with the ideal properties assumed in (4.7), there is another error term, v_{it}, that may be correlated with displacement:

$$(4.16) \quad y_{it} = \alpha_i + \gamma_t + x_{it}\beta + \sum_{k \geq -m} D_{it}^k \delta_k + v_{it} + \varepsilon_{it}.$$

To be concrete, suppose that a given worker can only be displaced at one particular date, say s, and that the probability of being displaced at date s depends only on the value of v_{is}. In this case, the nature of any biases that would be imparted to the estimates depends critically on the time series properties of the v_{it}.

At one extreme, $v_{i\tau}$ might be independent over time. In this case the only coefficient in (4.7) subject to any bias is δ_0. To see this, note that, according to (4.16),

$$(4.17) \quad E\,[y_{it} \mid i \text{ displaced at } s] = \alpha_i + \gamma_t + x_{it}\beta + \sum_{k \geq -m} D_{it}^k \delta_k + E\,[v_{it} \mid i$$
$$\text{displaced at } s].$$

If we let $\eta_{ts} = E[v_{it} \mid i$ displaced at $s]$, then the assumptions that displacement is influenced only by v_{is} and that the v_{it} are independent together imply that $\eta_{ts} = 0$ if $t \neq s$ and that

$$(4.18) \quad E\,[y_{it} \mid i \text{ displaced at } s] = \alpha_i + \gamma_t + x_{it}\beta + \sum_{k \geq -m} D_{it}^k \delta_k + D_{it}^0 \eta_{ss}.$$

Thus our estimator of the effect of displacement in the quarter in which it occurs tends toward $\delta_0 + \eta_{ss}$, rather than the true effect, δ_0. The other estimates will, however, be unaffected.

Unfortunately, when the v_{it} are correlated over time, bias in the estimators of the displacement effects is unlikely to be contained to δ_0. In general, just about any pattern of bias might arise. However, in the case where the v_{it} are a covariance stationary time series, some useful conclusions can be drawn. If the v_{it} are stationary, η_{ts} will depend only on the absolute value of the difference between t and s. That is, we can write $\eta_{ts} = \eta_{s-t}$ where $\eta_k = \eta_{-k}$. Thus when the v_{it} are a covariance stationary time series,

$$(4.19) \quad y_{it} = \alpha_i + \gamma_t + x_{it}\beta + \sum_{k \geq -m} D_{it}^k \delta_k + \sum_k D_{it}^k \eta_k + \varepsilon_{it}$$

where $\eta_k = \eta_{-k}$ and the ε_{it} are standard uncorrelated error terms. Thus, if firms displace workers when a stationary time series dips below a particular level at a certain date, a whole new set of "displacement effects" is introduced into the model of earnings determination. These effects are not associated with the true effect of displacement, but instead reflect the correlation between displacement and other unmeasured factors that affect earnings. When selection occurs on the basis of a stationary error term, there will be a form of statistical "bounceback" or "regression to the mean" that will occur after the separation independent of any true effects of displacement. These spurious displacement effects are, in general, nonzero for all k, but are constrained to be symmetric in the time relative to displacement.[18]

Most of the parameters in (4.19) are not identified. In particular, for $v \leq m$ we can only estimate $\delta_v - \delta_{-v}$. For $v > m$ we *can* identify δ_v because we can estimate η_{-v} from a version of our estimation procedure that includes dummies for each possible date relative to displacement (including those more than m periods before displacement). Given our assumption that $\delta_k = 0$ for $k < -m$, the coefficient on D_{it}^{-v} is an unbiased estimate of $\eta_{-v} = \eta_v$. On the other hand, the coefficient on D_{it}^{v} would be an unbiased estimate of $\delta_v + \eta_v$. Thus, subtracting one coefficient from the other would identify δ_v.[19]

We may recast the above discussion as an argument against the importance of the kind of bias induced by selection on a stationary error process for our estimates of the long-term effect of displacement. When we estimate our model allowing for displacement effects many periods prior to separation, we find no effects during the period more than three years before separation. Because the true and spurious effects of displacement are of the same sign, it follows that they must both be approximately zero. Moreover, when the error term is stationary, the spurious effects are symmetric about the date of displacement. Therefore, it follows that the bias we are discussing (the spurious effect of displacement) is also approximately zero more than three years after separation. Thus the biases resulting from displacement being related to low realizations of a stationary error term are unlikely to be important to our estimates of the long-run effects of displacement.

A more serious problem for estimating the earnings losses associated with displacement arises when the error in (4.7) is nonstationary. In this case, when firms discharge recent poor performers there is no reason to expect the earnings of those workers to recover. Had the discharged employees remained with their firms, their productivity or performance would have continued to be low. Therefore, it is unclear whether the estimated earnings losses result from the separation or from the fact that the employee had become a poor worker. We know of no way to modify our statistical model to resolve this question. Because we observe what is happening to the employment levels of the firm from which a worker is exiting, however, we can greatly diminish this source of bias. If a worker is leaving a firm at a time when many other workers are also separating, it is much more likely that the reasons for separation had to do with the impact of structural change on the firm and not the worker's unusually poor recent performance. Thus, in chapter 6 we focus on workers who were part of a mass layoff or plant closing. The earnings histories of that group of workers indicate that the foregoing concerns over selection bias are important.

4.4 Extensions of the Basic Model

The basic model described in section 4.2 meets one of the goals we set for our statistical specification—it displays the time pattern of losses due to displacement in a very flexible manner. However, as we have so far described it, it does not meet our other goal—that of summarizing how the losses associated with displacement vary across workers. In this section we describe how we have extended the basic model to achieve this second goal.

We want to be able to understand how the effects of displacement vary across groups of workers defined by such characteristics as sex, age, and industry of former employer. If the number of such categories is small, the most straightforward way to accomplish this is to include an entirely different set of δ_k's for each classification of worker:

$$(4.20) \quad y_{it} = \alpha_i + \gamma_t + x_{it}\beta + \sum_j \sum_{k \geq -m} E^j_{it} D^k_{it} \delta_{jk} + \varepsilon_{it}.$$

In (4.20), the various groups of workers are indexed by j and $E^j_{it} = 1$ if and only if worker i is in group j. The effect of displacement on a worker in the j'th category k periods after separation is given by δ_{jk}.

Estimating specification (4.20) is a feasible way to examine the differences in the effects of displacement between, say, men and women. In this case, the number of displacement parameters is only doubled. However, we also want to examine the relative size of the losses across relatively narrowly defined industry groupings and we also want to explore interactions in the sizes of losses between various factors. Thus the number of categories of workers we want to examine can become quite large, and basing our analysis on (4.20) would pose a computational problem and would require a good deal of effort simply to look at all the coefficients.[20]

In addition to employing (4.20) where it is feasible, we allow for variation in the effects of displacement across large numbers of categories of workers in a more parsimonious fashion. Specifically, we note that there are basically three important characteristics of the time pattern of displacement effects that differ across workers: (1) the rate at which earnings dip below their expected levels in the period before separation, (2) the size of the drop that occurs immediately after separation, and (3) the rate at which earnings recover. By allowing different categories of workers to differ on one parameter for each of these three characteristics of the time pattern, we obtain the relatively parsimonious specification (4.21):

$$(4.21) \quad y_{it} = \alpha_i + \gamma_t + x_{it}\beta + \sum_{k \geq -m} D_{it}^k \delta_k + \sum_j E_{it}^j (F_{it}^1 \varphi_{1j} + F_{it}^2 \varphi_{2j}$$

$$+ F_{it}^3 \varphi_{3j}) + \varepsilon_{it}.$$

In (4.21), F_{it}^1 and F_{it}^3 are time trends allowing for, respectively, different rates of decline before separation and different rates of recovery after separation. F_{it}^2 is a dummy variable allowing for different magnitudes of the drop occurring immediately after separation. More specifically,

$F_{it}^1 = t - (s - 13)$, if worker is displaced at time s and $s - 12 \leq t \leq s$

and $F_{it}^1 = 0$ otherwise.

$F_{it}^2 = 1$, if worker is displaced at time s and $t \geq s + 1$

and $F_{it}^2 = 0$ otherwise.

$F_{it}^3 = t - (s + 6)$, if worker is displaced at time s and $t \geq s+7$

and $F_{it}^3 = 0$ otherwise.

In terms of the parameterization of (4.21), the effect of displacement on a worker in the j'th category, k quarters after separation is

δ_k, if $k \geq \leq -12$.

$\delta_k + \varphi_{1j}(k + 13)$, if $-12 \leq k \leq 0$.

$\delta_k + \varphi_{2j}$, if $1 \leq k \leq 6$.

$\delta_k + \varphi_{2j} + \varphi_{3j}(k - 6)$, if $k \geq 7$.

Figure 4.2 depicts how the difference between the displacement effects of two different groups of workers is allowed to vary in (4.21). Specifically, up until 12 quarters prior to separation, the effects on earnings of the two groups is forced to be zero. From then until the actual separation, the two sets of estimates are allowed to diverge by an amount increasing linearly with time. At the date of actual separation, the two groups are allowed to drop by arbitrary amounts whose difference is assumed to be constant until six quarters after displacement. The effects on the two groups are then allowed to further diverge, again at a linear rate.

Figure 4.2 Difference Between Two Sets of Displacement Effect Estimates in Parsimonious Models

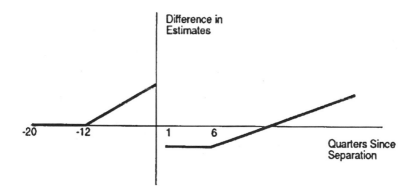

Specification (4.21) allows for a flexible but parsimonious form of variation across workers. It is also easily extended to allow for separate effects across two or more categories of workers without including all possible interactions. For instance, suppose that workers are categorized along a second dimension, indexed by q and represented with dummy variables, G_{it}^j. We can then allow the displacement effect to depend on both categorizations (those indexed by j and q) by employing the following specification:

$$(4.22) \quad y_{it} = \alpha_i + \gamma_t + x_{it}\beta + \sum_{k \geq -m} D_{it}^k \delta_k + \sum_j E_{it}^j (F_{it}^1 \varphi_{1j} + F_{it}^2 \varphi_{2j}$$

$$+ F_{it}^3 \varphi_{3j}) + \sum_q G_{it}^q (F_{it}^1 \varphi_{1j} + F_{it}^2 \varphi_{2j} + F_{it}^3 \varphi_{3j}).$$

In (4.22) both categorical variables determine the total effects of displacement in an additive manner. In chapter 6, we present estimates based on a model like (4.22), but with several factors interacting with the F_{it}^i variables. This allows us to determine, for example, how the effects of displacement differ between men and women, holding constant differences in industry and other factors.

So far, we have discussed how we can allow the displacement effects to vary across groups of workers. It is also informative in some cases to allow the coefficients on the control variables to vary across workers. For instance, we might want to allow for a different pattern of time effects for men and women. The means for accomplishing this goal parallel those for allowing the displacement effects to vary. If the number of categories is small, for example, we can simply allow for a completely different set of parameters for each category of workers. If a separate set of displacement effects is also included, it is then possible to simply estimate model (4.7) separately for each group. However, it is sometimes informative to allow for variation in the control coefficients over a large number of different categories of workers. When this is the case, we simply introduce a time trend specific to each category of worker, as in the following specification:

$$(4.23) \quad y_{it} = \alpha_i + \gamma_t + x_{it}\beta + \sum_j E_{it}^j T_{it} \lambda_j + \sum_{k \geq -m} D_{it}^k \delta_k$$

$$+ \sum_j E_{it}^j (F_{it}^1 \varphi_{1j} + F_{it}^2 \varphi_{2j} + F_{it}^3 \varphi_{3j}) + \varepsilon_{it}.$$

In (4.23), there is a separate time trend, $T_{it}\lambda_j$, for each group of worker. T_{it} might simply be time, or it might be time and time squared in which case λ_j would be a 2-vector of parameters. Specification (4.23) allows the earnings of certain groups of workers to be declining relative to others even if those workers are not displaced.

The danger in employing specifications such as (4.23) is, as we argued in section 4.1, that if the categories are defined too narrowly, we may miss the part of the displacement effect that is absorbed by all workers in an affected category rather than only by workers who actually lose their jobs. For instance, if the entire steel industry were affected by a reduction in import barriers and the effects of this impact was severely felt even by workers who kept their jobs, and, in addition, we had included in (4.23) a separate time trend for steel workers, we might obtain relatively small estimates of the displacement effects for this group. The reason would be that all steel workers were hurt and that the ones who actually lost their jobs were hurt only a little more. Nevertheless, we do report estimates of specifications such as (4.23). We do so because the differences between the estimates obtained using (4.22) and (4.23) with a large number of categories serve as indirect measures of the sizes of losses due to structural change that are imposed on workers who do not actually lose their jobs and because those differences shed some light on the nature of the earnings losses involved.

The final specification that we discuss goes beyond (4.23) by measuring earnings losses of displaced workers relative to the nondisplaced workers in their former firms. In specification (4.24), we introduce a complete set of interactions between the quarterly time effects, and indicators for the firms that workers were attached to in 1979 are introduced. If y_{ijt} denotes the earnings of worker i in 1979 firm j in quarter t, then

$$(4.24) \qquad y_{ijt} = \alpha_{ij} + \gamma_{jt} + \sum_{k \geq -m} D_{it}^k \delta_k + \varepsilon_{ijt} \quad .$$

If workers who retain their jobs in firms that lay off other workers also suffer earnings losses, then the γ_{jt}'s for those firms will decline around the time that layoffs occur and the estimates of the δ_k's will be closer to zero. The differences between displacement estimates obtained from (4.24) and (4.7) thus serve to gauge the size of losses suffered by workers who do not lose their jobs.

Specification (4.24) can only be estimated for the sample of displaced workers whose former firms remained in existence throughout the sample period. Therefore, estimates of this model necessarily exclude cases of complete firm closings.[21] However, estimation is straightforward. We simply calculate the mean for each quarter of the earnings of the workers who remained employed with their 1979 firms and subtract these means from the earnings of the workers who left the same firms. Displacement effects can then be calculated as in the second step of our two-step estimation procedure. (See equation (4.13).)

4.5 Conclusion

In this chapter, we developed a statistical framework for estimating the earnings losses of displaced workers. According to that framework workers' losses are measured by the difference between their actual earnings and their predicted earnings based on their own predisplacement earnings histories and the earnings histories of both other displaced and nondisplaced workers. Our model accounts explicitly for any fixed characteristics, both observed and unobserved, that affect earnings. Therefore, differences in the educational attainment, ethnicity, or innate ability among displaced and nondisplaced workers cannot account for the substantial earnings losses that we report in chapters 5 and 6. In addition, our model controls for the effect of time varying characteristics that are perfectly correlated with age. As a result, our estimated earnings losses are not caused by differing rates of earnings growth among workers of different ages.

Perhaps the most practical benefit of our framework is that it can easily account for how the average temporal pattern of losses varies with worker characteristics. While other studies have incorporated some of these features in their statistical frameworks, it has not been previously possible to implement a framework like ours, because the available data would not allow it. The reason that our framework can incorporate these features is because our administrative data enable us to construct long earnings histories for a large number of workers. Other longitudinal data sets such as the PSID or the NLS have too few observations on displacements to make our more comprehensive approach viable. Subsequent chapters present evidence of the feasibility of our framework for estimating the costs of worker dislocation.

NOTES

1. Another definition of the loss that might be appropriate in some circulstances is $E(y_{it} \mid D_{is} = 1) - E(y_{it})$. This definition compares displaced worker earnings to their unconditional expectation. It would presumably be even lower than (4.1) since the alternative to which displacement at date s is compared does not even rule out the possibility of displacement at date s.

2. The two quantities (and the measure mentioned in note 1) will be similar if the conditional probability is small. However, even among experienced, high-tenure workers, displacement was not a rare event in Pennsylvania in the 1980s. In fact, approximately 35 pecent of the workers in our sample separate from their firms.

3. As we have noted previously, our data set does not include such standard measures of accumulated human capital as years of education. As we explain in the next section, we exploit the longitudinal nature of the Pennsylvania data to make up for this lack of information on the demographics of the sample. The point here is that we want to allow the expectations in equation (4.5) to depend on the general characteristics of workers that help determine their earnings.

4. With a substantial amount of additional work, we would be able to condition on the establishment in which the worker was employed.

5. The literature on the costs to workers of structural change is perhaps already overly narrow in that it focuses only on workers who are actually forced to leave their firms. The use of measures such as (4.6) to compute the losses of displaced workers compounds this narrowness by focusing only on the loss associated with the actual separation.

6. When k is negative, $D_{it}^{k} = 1$ if the worker was displaced $\mid k \mid$ periods after period t.

7. See section 4.3 for a discussion of the consequences of not allowing for a correlation of a_i with D_{it}^{k}.

8. Of course, (4.13) can also be made computationally tractable by taking deviations from means. Many of the actual computations reported below were made by invoking the ABSORB statement of PROC GLM in SAS which automates the deviation from means technique.

9. This is not surprising. Most of the information in the data relevant to estimating β and the γ_t's is pretty clearly contained in the data for the nondisplaced workers. It is also worth noting that (4.7) can be estimated without using any data on nondisplaced workers. In effect, different cohorts of displaced workers can act as comparison groups for each other. However, doing the estimation without the nondisplaced workers greatly increases the uncertainty in the estimates of β and the γ_t's and this uncertainty is largely transferred to the δ_k's. Adding the data on the nondisplaced workers tightly pins down β and the γ_t's and allows the data on the displaced workers to much more precisely estimate the δ_k's.

10. Alternatively, $\sum D_{it}^{k} = 1$ for displaced workers for all t. Similarly, the sum of the worker-specific dummy variable implicit in (4.7) is also always equal to 1. This equality demonstrates linear dependence among the columns of the design underlying (4.7) and thus lack of identification in the case where we have no data on displaced workers prior to m quarters before their displacement.

11. Increasing m decreases the precision of our estimates since it effectively reduces the number of worker-quarter observations that go into computing the estimate of normal, predisplacement earnings of displaced workers. This effect is not, however, very pronounced in the range of m we have used.

12. That is, the effects of displacement would appear more negative than they actually were. This assumes that workers with low regular earnings are more likely to be displaced. If workers with high regular earnings were more likely to be displaced, the bias would be in the other direction.

13. We are assuming that the means were all based on data from the same calendar quarter and that the two groups of workers had the same means for the variables included in x_{it}.

14. Actually, since quarter dummies are also included in the model, pure time series variation in earnings is also irrelevant to the estimation of the model.

15. That is, the estimates would tend to show the effects of displacement as being bigger in absolute value than they are in reality.

16. Model (4.14) could also be estimated by computing regressions on various kinds of second-differenced data just as (4.7) could be estimated by computing regressions on first-differenced data.

17. See Jacobson, LaLonde, and Sullivan (1992).

18. If specific parametric assumptions on the time series of errors, such as that they follow a low-order moving average or autoregressive process, were adopted, then the dependence of the η_k on k could be further restricted and, perhaps, be used as the basis for an estimation strategy that corrects for the effects of selection.

19. See Heckman and Robb (1985) for a similar argument in support of the use of a "symmetric difference in differences" estimator in the program evaluation context.

20. Admittedly, the computational problems are not terribly severe. This is especially true if the two-step estimation technique is applied. That is, in the first stage the nondisplaced workers can be used to estimate β and the γ_t's. With these subtracted from the earnings data of the displaced workers, (4.20) can be estimated separately for each category of worker. The problem of absorbing the information in all the coefficients remains, however.

21. Actually, we need the slightly stronger criterion that the firm continued to have workers who were in our sample of nondisplaced workers.

5
Earnings Losses Associated
With Worker Separations

In the previous chapter, we argued that earnings losses of displaced workers should be defined as the difference between workers' actual earnings and the earnings they would have received had the events that led to their displacements never occurred. According to this definition, the displacement effect is potentially larger than the earnings change from immediately before their separations. Our framework allows for the possibility that the events leading to separations cause earnings to decline even before workers leave their firms. These pre-separation losses may result from reductions in overtime hours, real wage cuts, or temporary layoffs.

In this chapter, we estimate the temporal pattern of these earnings losses for a sample of prime-age, high-tenure workers who separated from their firms between 1980 and 1986. As discussed in chapter 3, we limit our analysis to these workers partly out of a desire to focus on the losses of high-tenure workers, and partly to mitigate the problems associated with distinguishing among quits, retirements, and layoffs in administrative data. In addition, our sample includes only workers who remain attached to Pennsylvania's wage and salary workforce. As a result, the substantial long-term earnings losses reported in this chapter do not result from prolonged periods of nonemployment. Indeed, it is reduced hours or reduced real wages on new jobs that are the primary causes of these losses.

Table 5.1 presents mean 1979 age and earnings for our samples of separators and nondisplaced workers. As shown in Panel A of the table, the median age of the separators is 37, and 80 percent are between the ages of 27 and 47. This mean age and range also characterizes the ages of the nondisplaced workers in the sample. As a result, we describe the sample as being made up largely of prime-age adults. Further, this characterization of workers' ages holds for several groups in the sample, namely, male and female workers, workers from different geographical regions and industrial sectors, and workers separating from firms that may have experienced a mass layoff or plant closing.

The earnings figures in the bottom panel of table 5.1 indicate that the median separator earned $22,904 (1987 dollars) in 1979, or about $2,000 less than the median worker in our sample of nondisplaced workers. Further, with the exception of the females in the sample, the other separator groups received approximately the same earnings. Despite being nearly the same age, the separators earned about 9 percent less than nondisplaced, workers. That fact indicates that less skilled workers are more likely to be displaced, and without properly controlling for this skills disparity, we might overstate the losses associated with displacement. The statistical framework developed in chapter 4 addresses this disparity by incorporating individual "fixed effects" into the model.

Below we present our estimates of the earnings losses connected with the events that lead to job separations. Following equation (4.7), we report the estimated parameters associated with separation status of workers for each quarter beginning with the 20th quarter prior to their separations and ending with the 27th quarter after their separations. The precision with which we can estimate these parameters varies with the time relative to separation.[1] On the one hand, because every worker in the sample has earnings histories that begin more than five years before the first workers separate from their firms, data on all separators' earnings directly contribute to estimating the 20 preseparation parameters. During this period, the standard errors associated with our estimates average $30 per quarter. On the other hand, we only observe earnings six years after separations if workers left their former firms during 1980. Thus, it is this group of workers who largely determine the long-term effects of separation. Because these long-term estimates are based on a smaller sample of separators, they are less precise than the preseparation and short-term postseparation estimates. Accordingly, by the 20th quarter after separations, the standard errors associated with our estimates have risen to $60 per quarter.

Table 5.1 Sample Characteristics

Workers	Observations	Mean	Standard deviation	Median	10th percentile	90th percentile
Panel A: 1979 Age						
Separators						
All	9,507	37.0	7.4	37	27	47
Males	7,092	36.9	7.2	37	27	47
Females	2,415	37.3	7.8	38	27	48
Nonmanufacturing	2,870	36.9	7.3	37	27	47
Manufacturing	6,637	37.1	7.4	37	27	47
Western Pennsylvania	3,804	36.8	7.4	37	27	47
Eastern Pennsylvania	5,703	37.1	7.3	37	27	47
Nonmass layoffs	3,072	36.9	7.3	37	27	47
Mass layoffs	6,435	37.1	7.4	37	27	47
Stayers	13,704	37.7	7.0	38	28	47
Panel B: 1979 Earnings (1987 dollars)						
Separators						
All	9,507	$24,196	$12,287	$22,904	$11,525	$36,798
Males	7,092	27,363	12,161	25,942	16,326	38,557
Females	2,415	14,897	6,641	14,275	7,595	22,928
Nonmanufacturing	2,870	24,648	15,547	22,363	10,029	39,358
Manufacturing	6,637	24,001	10,566	23,096	12,070	35,963

88

Table 5.1 Sample Characteristics

Workers	Observations	Mean	Standard deviation	Median	10th percentile	90th percentile
Western Pennsylvania	3,804	$25,147	$12,449	$24,292	$12,359	$37,561
Eastern Pennsylvania	5,703	23,561	12,138	22,176	11,005	36,140
Nonmass layoffs	3,072	23,640	14,415	21,665	10,585	36,726
Mass layoffs	6,435	24,461	11,120	23,593	12,037	36,805
Stayers	13,704	26,322	12,980	24,867	13,644	38,880

5.1 Earnings Losses For Workers Who Separate From Their Firms

This study indicates that earnings of high-tenure workers decline substantially when they separate from their firms. As shown by figure 5.1, approximately three years prior to their separations, quarterly earnings of such workers begin to diverge from their expected levels. That divergence accelerates as separations approach. In the quarter immediately prior to separation, earnings depart from their predicted levels by approximately $750. When workers leave their firms, their quarterly earnings fall sharply, and one year after their separation, earnings remain $1,500 below their expected levels. More significantly, five years after separation, their earnings remain $1,000 per quarter below their expected levels, an amount equal to 20 percent of their preseparation earnings.

Figure 5.1 Earnings Losses of High-Attachment Separators

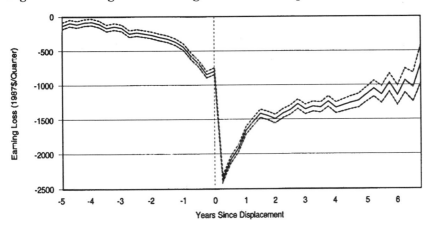

Estimate and 95% Confidence Interval Shown

Figure 5.1 also reveals that after workers separate from their firms, their earnings recover at a modest rate. Between one and six years following their separations, earnings of these workers increase by approximately $30 per quarter relative to their expected levels. Should that rate of growth continue, their earnings would equal their expected earnings approximately 14 years after separation. At a discount rate of 4 percent, that rate of convergence suggests that job separations cost the typical high-tenure worker approximately $50,000.

The substantial earnings losses observed in figure 5.1 are largely due to reduced earnings in new jobs rather than simply increased time spent unemployed. As shown by figure 5.2, the quarterly employment rates of these workers only depart substantially from their expected levels during the first year following separation. After this period, quarterly employment rates of separators are only 3 or 4 percent less than their predicted levels. This finding is not surprising as our sample excludes workers with extremely long spells without wage and salary earnings. Indeed, one reason we study these particular workers is that any ensuing earnings losses are largely the result of real wage cuts or hour reductions on a new job and not of long unemployment spells.

Figure 5.2 Employment Probability Losses of High-Attachment Separators

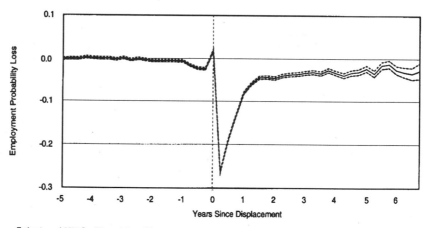

Estimate and 95% Confidence Interval Shown

Our confidence in the findings presented in figure 5.1 is strengthened by the pattern of preseparation earnings losses. One informal test of our specification (4.7) is that earnings should equal their expected earnings several years prior to separation. As seen in figure 5.1, the separation effect is not meaningful until three to four years before workers leave their jobs. Prior to that time,   actual and expected earnings nearly coincide. To further explore this point, we examine the differences between actual and expected preseparation earnings for workers who left their firms after 1983. This group's preseparation earnings data cover a 10-year period. Our analysis indicates that their earnings equaled their expected earnings for over seven years before diverging during the three years prior to separation.[2] These findings suggest that our econometric framework is not overly restrictive, and that any systematic differences between trend rate of earnings growth for separators and stayers are likely to be small.

In this study, we consistently find that workers experience substantial earnings losses prior to actually leaving the firm.[3] As noted above, in the quarter prior to separation, earnings are already $750 below their expected levels. That figure is slightly less than the estimated earnings loss six years after separation. One interpretation of this finding is that displaced workers suffer only modest long-term losses. Because their losses prior to leaving their jobs are not much smaller than their losses after six years, their earnings have, in effect, nearly returned not only to preseparation levels, but to the levels they would have expected to receive after six years just prior to leaving their former jobs.

This interpretation underscores the importance of the distinctions made in chapter 4 between different definitions of displaced worker earnings losses. Those definitions depend on when during workers' earnings histories we calculated their expected earnings. The evidence of increased earnings losses during the preseparation period suggests that workers have reason to expect lower future earnings even prior to their job losses.

In chapter 3 we discussed why our results might show that earnings of displaced workers decline prior to their job losses. One possibility was that, because in some cases we may date separations after they actually occur, what we identify as preseparation losses might really result from postseparation earnings declines. However, we do not believe this explanation to be very compelling. First, we probably do not miss the actual date by more than a few quarters, and the decline in earnings begins at least three years before separation. Second, in our analysis below we find that preseparation earnings losses depend on sex and industry of workers, and on the economic well-being of their former firms. Women and nonmanufacturing workers, as well as workers separating from stable or growing firms, experience substantially smaller predisplacement losses than other groups. While dating separations may remain a problem, we do not see why it should be a more difficult problem for men and manufacturing workers, or for workers separating from firms that have experienced mass layoffs.

Rather, we believe that the preseparation earnings losses we observe are a real phenomenon resulting from decisions of firms to cut real wages, reduce overtime hours, or temporarily lay off workers before they permanently lay them off. Unfortunately, because administrative data do not report wages or hours, we cannot determine the importance of wage cuts or lost overtime. However, we can use our data to explore the importance of the increased incidence of temporary layoffs. It is already apparent from figure 5.2 that because employment rates of displaced workers remain high prior to worker separation, layoffs lasting an entire quarter cannot account for much of the predisplacement earnings losses. By examining data on receipt of unemployment insurance (UI) benefits we can examine whether relatively short layoffs explain much of the magnitude of these losses.

Temporary layoffs are not uncommon among our samples of displaced and nondisplaced workers. Even during the late 1970s, when workers in both of these samples remained employed with the same firm, they would occasionally experience spells of insured unemployment. For example, during 1977 through 1979, UI receipts of nondisplaced workers averaged $27 per quarter. However, when displaced workers approached their separation dates, their UI receipts rose above these normal levels. As shown by figure 5.3, we find that UI receipts rise one year prior to job separation and peak one quarter after separation. Not surprisingly, as shown by figure 5.4, that same pattern holds for the number of weeks during the quarter that displaced workers received UI benefits. The two figures indicate that one quarter prior to the quarters of separation, unemployment benefits and weeks of receipts for subsequently displaced workers were $150 and 0.75 weeks, respectively, above their expected levels.

Figure 5.3 Excess Unemployment Insurance and Trade Adjustment Assistance Benefits of High-Attachment Separators

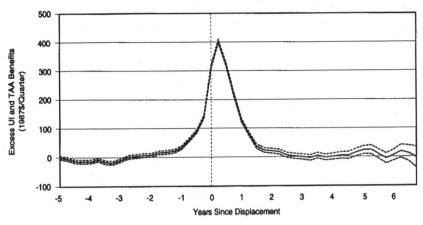

Estimate and 95% Confidence Interval Shown

Figure 5.4 Excess Weeks of Unemployment Insurance and Trade Adjustment Assistance Claims of High-Attachment Separators

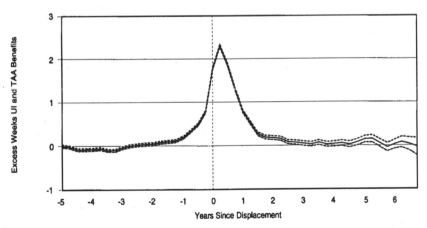

Estimate and 95% Confidence Interval Shown

We may use the findings in figure 5.3 and figure 5.4 to estimate what the earnings of separators would have been had they not been laid off. If we assume that the UI replacement rate for these high-tenure workers is 40 percent, the benefits they receive should constitute approximately 40 percent of their regular earnings. In light of this assumption, we estimate that earnings losses would have been $375 less in the quarter prior to their separations had there been no temporary layoffs. These calculations suggest that temporary layoffs may account for approximately one-half of preseparation quarterly earnings losses.[4]

The data on receipt of UI benefits also helps us to isolate a group of separators whom we are sure left their jobs because they were laid off. Because of the long and continuous earnings histories of separators, anyone who was laid off was certainly eligible to receive UI benefits. Thus, it is not surprising that whether a worker received UI benefits after separation is an important predictor of the temporal pattern of his or her earnings losses. As shown by figure 5.5, the entire pattern of losses differs between those who collected and those who did not collect UI benefits. During the preseparation period, only those who subsequently collected UI benefits experienced large earnings losses. During the postseparation period, those who collected UI benefits experienced long-term losses amounting to more than $1,500 per quarter. Those separators who did not collect experienced much smaller losses, but their quarterly earnings remained approximately $600 below their expected levels throughout most of the postseparation period. These smaller losses for the non-UI collectors are consistent with this group being an amalgam of workers who left their former jobs because they quit, were discharged for cause, were laid off and immediately found a new job, or were laid off and simply did not collect.

As Blank and Card (1990) observe, not everyone who appears to be eligible to receive UI benefits files a claim to receive these benefits. Anderson and Meyer (1992) have found as we have, in similar administrative data that even following mass layoffs, less than 50 percent of experienced workers ever collect benefits. One reason may be that some workers find new jobs soon after their separations. In support of that argument, we could find only a few instances in which separators who did not collect any UI benefits had a quarter with zero earnings following their separations. Therefore, one problem with studying the losses of displaced persons who received UI benefits is that we are focusing on the group that is having the most difficult time adjusting to job loss. As a result, their earnings losses likely over-state the average costs of worker displacement. Nonetheless, the gap between the earnings losses of UI collectors and noncollectors indicates that the estimates presented earlier in figure 5.1 result from the adverse experiences of displaced workers.

Figure 5.5 Earnings Losses for Unemployment Insurance Benefit Collectors and Noncollectors

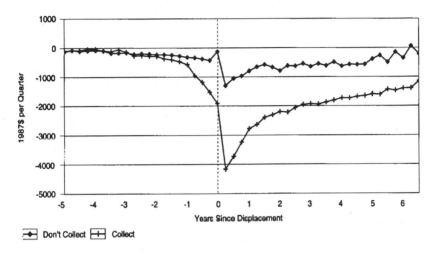

5.2 Earnings Losses and the Comparison Group

As discussed in chapter 4, earnings loss estimates may depend on who is chosen to be in the comparison group. The comparison group's composition is important because earnings growth may differ across firms or sectors. In the foregoing analysis, the comparison group consisted of workers hired before 1974 who remained with their firms through 1986. Their earnings growth identified the impact of age and macroeconomic factors on earnings. By constructing our comparison group the way we did, we implicitly compared separators to the typical nonseparator. In other words, the earnings loss estimates express how workers' earnings performed relative to their own past earnings histories and relative to workers who remained at the average firm (when weighted by size).

Alternatively, it is of interest to know how earnings of separators performed relative to nonseparators from their own former firms. For example, the estimated earnings losses based on this estimator should be smaller if the earnings of those who stay in firms that discharge large fractions of their workforces are depressed compared with the earnings of those who stay in firms that discharge few employees. The difference between these two sets of estimates is indicative of the losses suffered by nonseparators when fellow employees leave their firms.

In chapter 4, we showed that using a comparison group made up of nondisplaced workers from separators' former firms amounts to adding to our model (4.7) interactions between the model's time effects and an indicator of workers' firms. These interactions imply that the time effects are identified not merely by the impact of macroeconomic conditions on statewide earnings, but by the impact of these conditions on average earnings of individual firms. One drawback of this procedure is that we must estimate losses for a different sample of separators, because firms that close have no corresponding comparison group. Therefore, the earnings loss estimates based on the alternative comparison group are only for separators who leave firms that remain open throughout the sample period.

For this group of separators, figure 5.6 displays loss estimates using model (4.7), which is equivalent to using the typical stayer as a comparison group and using model (4.24), which is equivalent to using a separate comparison group made up of the stayers in the worker's own firm for each separator. As the figure shows, changing the comparison group to include only stayers in the separator's former firm reduces the estimated earnings losses by about 25 percent. Five years after their separations, quarterly earnings of workers are $900 below their expected levels after controlling for the time pattern of earnings growth in their former firms. In contrast, the loss estimates for the corresponding group without such firm controls are $1,200. Nonetheless, no matter which comparison group is preferred, the estimated earnings losses associated with separations remain substantial.

It is also worth noting that the difference between the two loss estimates shown in figure 5.6 can be taken as an estimate of the losses suffered by workers who keep their jobs in firms in which others separate, relative to the typical worker who remains with a single firm throughout the period. As the figure indicates, even the nondisplaced workers in separators' former firms experience some modest earnings declines.

Figure 5.6 Earnings Losses of High-Attachment Separators from Surviving Firms Relative to All Stayers and Relative to Stayers in Their Former Firms

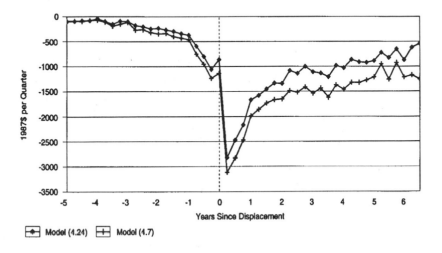

Another important point illustrated by the estimates shown in figure 5.6 for the comparison with stayers in separators' former firms is that the factors that cause earnings to decline prior to separation do not equally affect all employees in the firm. That is, because the pre-separation earnings loss estimates do not depend significantly on which comparison group we use, they must result from earnings of separators falling substantially relative to similar workers from the same firms. As shown by figure 5.6, three years prior to separation, earnings nearly coincided with expected earnings based on the experiences of other workers in their firms. However, during the year prior to separation, their earnings diverge significantly from expected levels. This implies that the earnings of nondisplaced workers in the firm are not as adversely affected by the events that eventually lead to separations of others as are the earnings of those who actually separate. This finding suggests that when firms reduce their workforces, it probably becomes apparent well before workers permanently leave who these separators are likely to be. Our findings on the preseparation receipt of UI benefits suggest that workers on temporary layoff are those most likely to be permanently laid off at a later date.

5.3 Earnings Losses by Gender, Industrial Sector, Age, and Region

The same pattern of earnings losses that held for the full sample of workers also holds within different demographic groups and for workers separating from firms in different industrial sectors and regions of the state. Specifically, earnings losses arise prior to separations and remain substantial following separations. However, the relative magnitudes of these effects do differ somewhat across groups.

For example, as shown by figure 5.7, both women and men experience substantial earnings losses when they separate from their firms. Six years following separations, quarterly earnings of both men and women are $1,000 and $1,500, respectively, below their expected levels. Because men's preseparation earnings averaged $6,400 per quarter, and women's preseparation earnings averaged $3,700 per quarter, in percentage terms men's losses are actually slightly smaller than women's losses.

There are, however, two noteworthy differences between the patterns of earnings losses of women and men. First, the preseparation earnings declines for women are smaller than for men. Women's preseparation earnings only begin to depart significantly from their expected levels two years before leaving their firms. By comparison, men's earnings begin $200 below their expected levels, decline more than three years prior to leaving their jobs, and fall at a faster rate. Second, women's postseparation earnings decline by much less than men's but also recover at a much slower rate. In fact, there is little evidence that women's earnings are recovering at all beyond two years following their separations. By contrast, after the second year following separation, men's earnings approach their expected levels at a rate of approximately $40 per quarter. At that rate of recovery, men's earnings would return to their expected levels 14 years after separation.

Figure 5.7 Earnings Losses of Male and Female High-Attachment Separators

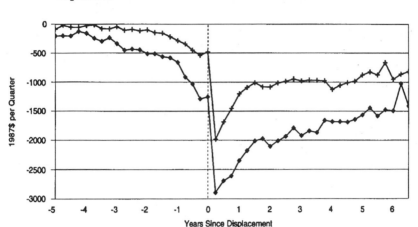

The differences between earnings loss patterns of women and men partly reflect the industries in which they work. As shown in figure 5.8, workers separating from both the nonmanufacturing and manufacturing sectors experience substantial earnings losses. But, the losses in the nonmanufacturing sector, where women are more likely to work, are substantially smaller prior to separation and diverge significantly from their expected levels only in the last year before separation. After leaving their firms, the earnings of nonmanufacturing workers fall less sharply and recover more slowly relative to their expected levels than do the earnings of manufacturing workers.

Workers' ages at the time of separation also appear to be a modest determinant of their earnings losses. But more significantly, we find that high-tenure workers of all ages incur substantial long-term earnings losses when they separate from their firms. As shown by figure 5.9, five years after separation, even the quarterly earnings of the youngest group of workers who were less than 30 years old in 1979 remain $800 below their expected levels. The earnings of these workers recover at a modest rate after their separations. Beginning with the second year following separation, their earnings approach the expected levels at a rate of $54 per quarter. At that rate of recovery, the earnings of these younger workers would return to their expected levels within nine years after their separations.

Figure 5.8 Earnings Losses of Manufacturing and Nonmanufacturing High-Attachment Separators

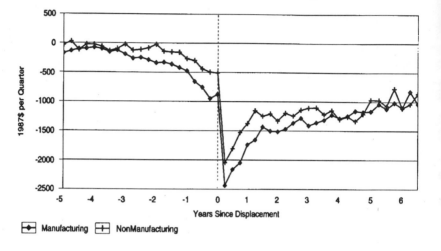

Older workers experience somewhat larger losses. More important, however, we find little evidence that their earnings will ever return to their expected levels. The quarterly earnings of workers who were between 40 and 50 years old in 1979 remain nearly $1,500 below their expected levels. That loss is approximately the same in the fifth year as it was in the second year following separation. Taken together, these results for older and younger workers do not necessarily indicate that older workers fare worse following displacements than their younger counterparts. Although, both of these groups include only high-tenure workers, the older workers probably had more years of service when they separated from their firms than did the younger workers. Therefore, the earnings losses we observe for different birth cohorts are due to the combined effects of tenure and age on earnings losses.

**Figure 5.9 Earnings Losses of 1930s, 1940s, and 1950s Birth Cohort
High-Attachment Separators**

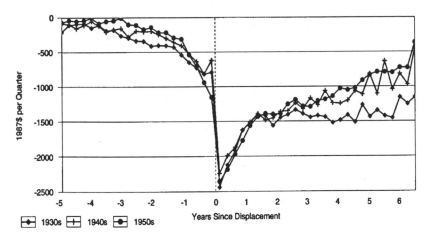

Finally, the condition of labor markets appears to be a determinant of earnings losses. Although workers in both the state's eastern and western halves experienced substantial losses when they separated from their firms, the losses were larger among workers separating from firms in the state's western section. As shown by figure 5.10, the long-term quarterly earnings losses amount to approximately $1,500 in the state's western half, where unemployment rates were high during the early and mid-1980s. In contrast, those losses were only $800 in the state's eastern half, where by the mid-1980s unemployment rates in some places had fallen below 6 percent. The patterns of relatively small preseparation earnings declines and slower-than-average postseparation earnings recoveries in the state's eastern half are consistent with its smaller share of manufacturing employment. However, we have found that even among workers displaced from Pennsylvania's manufacturing firms, those from the state's western section incurred larger losses than those from manufacturing firms in the eastern section of the state.

Figure 5.10 Earnings Losses of Eastern and Western Pennsylvania High-Attachment Separators

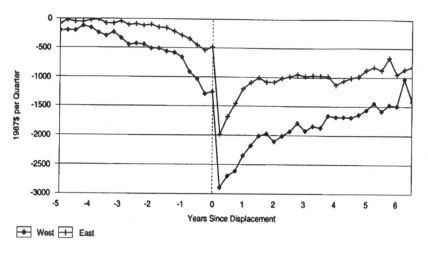

5.4 Conclusions

This chapter documents that when high-tenure prime-age workers separate from their firms they incur substantial long-term earnings losses. We find that their annual earnings are approximately $4,000, or roughly 17 percent, below their expected levels even five to six years after leaving their former firms. In addition, we find that these earnings losses first appear even before workers leave their firms. This pattern of losses appears to hold for workers from different demographic groups, sectors, and regions. Finally, these findings are only modestly affected by whether we use a comparison group made up of all nondisplaced workers in the state or only of nondisplaced workers from the separators' former firms. To be sure, the loss estimates are approximately 25 percent smaller when we use nondisplaced workers from their former firms as the comparison group. That difference suggests that the events leading to separations also adversely affect those who remain behind. Both sets indicate that large losses persist, however.

We find the foregoing pattern of losses even though our sample of separators may include workers who quit or were discharged for cause from their former jobs. Because we have a representative sample of prime-age, high-tenure workers during that period, it is clear that for these workers separations lead, on average, to lower earnings. What is not so clear is whether this pattern of losses characterizes the pattern for workers who separate involuntarily from their firms for economic reasons. We believe our sample's composition with its high fraction of older, high-tenure workers implies that most separators are, in fact, leaving their firms because of economic restructuring. However, because the study has not specifically singled out such workers, it remains possible that our findings are an amalgamation for three distinct groups. Persons discharged for cause may also experience earnings losses. But for that group the losses do not reflect events adversely affecting the firm. Instead, they reflect poor employee performance.[5] Finally, employees who quit would not necessarily experience earnings losses. Those who quit presumably are moving into better and more highly paid jobs. In the next chapter we show how our findings hold up when we distinguish more precisely among these groups of separators.

NOTES

1. It is useful to include data on workers separating in the latter years in our sample period, even if our only interest were in the long-term effect of separations. Clearly, the postseparation experiences of the workers who separate in the early 1980s directly contribute to our understanding of long-term losses, but those experiences also determine our estimates of the relative size of short- and long-term losses. Thus, the information contributed by workers displaced in the mid-1980s, which directly helps estimate short-term losses, when combined with information on the relative severity of short- and long-term losses, helps estimate the long-term losses.

2. Because our earnings histories begin in 1974, only those separating during or after 1984 have preseparation earnings covering a 10-year period.

3. Two recent studies report preseparation wage losses among displaced workers in both the DWS and in the PSID. Di la Rica (1992) using an estimation strategy similar to that used by Seitchik and Zornitsky (1989) as described in chapter 2. She reports that displaced workers in the 1986 DWS incurred preseparations earnings losses that amounted to 11 percent of their wages. Ruhm (1991a), using a differencing framework and a comparison group, reports that displaced workers in the PSID incurred preseparations earnings losses of 6 to 10 percent of their wages.

4. Ruhm (1991a, pp. 171-72) reports a similar result using the PSID. From the second to the first year prior to their displacements, workers report that their time spent unemployed increases by approximately 1.5 weeks.

5. This situation is captured by the model developed in chapter 4, when the errors follow a random walk. In that instance, a decline in employee productivity would be permanent.

6
Earnings Losses
and Mass Layoffs

The previous chapter examined the earnings losses that arise when high-tenure workers separate from their firms. That examination did not distinguish, however, among the circumstances that lead to employee separations. By restricting our sample to high-tenure workers born after 1930, we tried to reduce the interpretive difficulties associated with the possibility that some separations result from quits and retirements. In spite of that effort, some separators in the sample may have left their jobs for those reasons or may have been discharged for cause. These distinctions are potentially important as subsequent labor market performance of workers may depend on the circumstances under which they left their former firms. For example, the postseparation earnings of those who quit their former jobs may differ from those who were laid off because of demand shifts or technology changes. In the former instance, earnings are likely to rise, while in the latter instance earnings are likely to decline. These considerations suggest that the previous chapter's estimated earnings losses may provide a misleading picture of the temporal pattern of earnings losses associated with worker dislocation.

In this chapter, we analyze how the circumstances surrounding worker separations relate to the pattern of their losses by examining the relationship between their earnings losses and the economic health of their firms at the time of separation. We measure the economic health of firms by the change in their employment. We define distressed firms as those whose employment declined by more than 30 percent from their late-1970s peak. This category includes firms that closed as well as those that experienced mass layoffs. Presumably, most separators from this mass layoff subsample left involuntarily and for reasons unrelated to their performance.[1] Alternatively, our nonmass layoff subsample consists of workers from growing firms as well as those from firms whose employment fell by less than

30 percent. This subsample probably includes a larger share of workers who quit their jobs or were dismissed for cause.

In the next section, we examine directly the relationship between earnings losses of workers and the economic health of their firm. In section 6.2, we examine the relationship between those earnings losses and our choice of a comparison group. One concern in that section is whether nondisplaced workers in distressed firms also experience earnings losses. In section 6.3, we examine how the temporal pattern of earnings losses varies among workers in several broadly defined industries. In section 6.4, we implement a more parsimonious version of our model to examine how the pattern of losses varies among industries defined by their 1- or 2-digit SIC codes. In sections 6.5 and 6.6 we show how earnings losses vary according to gender and age of workers and their local labor market conditions. Finally, in section 6.7, we examine how those losses depend on whether displaced workers from distressed firms find new jobs that are similar to their old jobs.

6.1 Relation Between Worker and Firm Fortunes

Our definition of a distressed firm isolates employees associated with firms that experienced mass layoffs or plant closings during the early and mid-1980s. Although some employees from that sample may have quit their jobs for financial or personal reasons or were discharged for cause, the vast majority probably involuntarily separated from their firms for economic reasons. Further, because fewer workers discharged during mass layoffs are likely to be marginal employees, this subsample of separators may include workers for whom the employment relationship was especially valuable.

Figure 6.1 shows how earnings losses vary with the level of employment change of separators' firms. The estimates are based on specification (4.20), in which a completely different set of displacement effects is estimated for each of four firm classes. In each case, however, the losses are relative to expected earnings based on the experiences of all nonseparators. As the figure shows, workers displaced as a part of large reductions in their firms' workforces experience substantially larger earnings losses than other employees who separate from their firms. As indicated by the two lower lines in the figure, quarterly earnings of such employees decline by $1,000 relative to their expected earnings prior to their displacements. That decline is substantially larger than the decline experienced by other discharged employees.[2] After their displacements, the earnings of employees from distressed firms fall by another $2,000 below their expected levels. After recovering rapidly during the first postdisplacement year, quarterly earnings remain between $1,000 and $2,000 below their predicted levels. These long-term losses equal approximately 25 percent of predisplacement earnings.

Figure 6.1 Earnings Losses by Difference Between Employment Level of Firm at Time of Separation and 1974-1979 Maximum

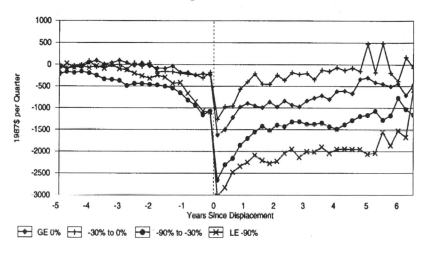

In contrast to employees who separate from distressed firms, those separating from stable firms experience substantially smaller earnings losses. As shown by the second highest line in figure 6.1, this group's earnings prior to separation were only $250 below their expected levels. Following separation, earnings fell $1,500 below their expected levels. That earnings gap declines with time, but after six years, it remains at $500 per quarter. This finding of a permanent loss for workers separating from stable firms suggests that most workers in this subsample probably did not separate from their firms because they quit their jobs. If most of these separators had quit their jobs, it would be odd that, on average, those quits led to lower earnings.

It is possible that many separators in stable firms probably neither quit nor were laid off for economic reasons, but were discharged for poor performance. The findings in figure 6.1 suggest that such discharges are associated with long-term losses. Indeed, it is not surprising that job losses resulting from common reasons for dismissal such as productivity declines, excessive absenteeism, or substance abuse would lead to substantial earnings losses. Moreover, these causes for discharge would be associated with small preseparation earnings losses as long as employees' quarterly earnings did not generally reflect variations in their own quarterly productivity. As that relationship is not likely to be particularly strong for this sample of workers, it is not surprising that the preseparation earnings losses would be small.[3] Of course, because we cannot distinguish with much confidence among the reasons for worker separations, these findings are merely suggestive of the potential losses associated with discharges for cause.

Further evidence that earnings losses depend on the circumstances under which employees separate from their firms is seen in the losses experienced by workers who leave firms experiencing modest employment declines. Firms might prefer to first lay off workers who in the future would be less costly to replace, and such workers are more likely to be marginal employees than workers separating from distressed firms. As a result, we expect small earnings losses when firms lay off only a few workers. Indeed, as shown by figure 6.1, prior to their separations, earnings losses of those workers are the same as of employees leaving stable firms. After their separations, their earnings approach expected levels within one year and recover within five years. For this group there appears to be no long-term earnings loss associated with their separations.

6.2 Earnings Losses and the Comparison Group

We observed in section 5.2 that estimates of earnings losses experienced by separators were smaller when we compared their earnings to those of the nonseparators from their former firms. We show below that those lower loss estimates result from differences between the earnings growth of nondisplaced workers in distressed and nondistressed firms. To arrive at this result we analyze the losses of workers leaving distressed firms separately from those of workers leaving stable or modestly declining firms. Figure 6.2 shows loss estimates obtained using both comparison groups for workers from distressed firms. The figure indicates that the long-term earnings losses for workers separating from distressed firms decline from approximately $1,500 per quarter to approximately $1,200 per quarter when we change from using all stayers to only stayers from workers' former firms as the comparison group. Alternatively, the difference between the two earnings loss measures indicates that the earnings of nondisplaced workers in distressed firms declined permanently by approximately $300 per quarter relative to the average nondisplaced worker.

The foregoing findings show that structural change adversely affects both displaced and nondisplaced workers. The adverse effects on those who keep their jobs are only one-fifth as large as on those who lose them. Nevertheless, estimated losses based on the earnings of former co-workers who remain employed clearly understate the full loss to displaced workers associated with the events that bring about their job losses. Such estimates only measure the impact of job loss *per se* and do not take into account the simultaneous earnings declines for the nondisplaced workers in their former firms. Because we are most interested in the question of the importance to the fortunes of workers of the events that lead to displacement, in what follows we emphasize estimated losses based on a comparison group of all nondisplaced workers.

Our interpretation of the difference between the earnings loss measures depicted in figure 6.2 is supported by the similarity between these measures shown in figure 6.3 for workers separating from growing or modestly declining firms. The earnings loss estimates for these separators are unaffected by our choice of a comparison group. As shown by figure 6.3, no matter which comparison group is used, earnings losses of these workers are small prior to their separations, large during the first year after their separations, but recover in the long term. Not surprisingly, these findings indicate that when only a few employees separate from their firms, those separations are not associated with losses for workers who remain at the old firm.

110

Figure 6.2 Earnings Losses Relative to Typical Nondisplaced Worker (Model (4.7)) and Relative to Workers in Displaced Workers' Former Firms (Model (4.24)): Workers in Distressed but Surviving Firms

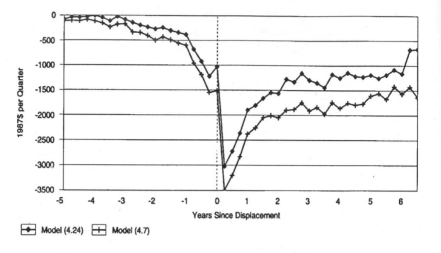

Figure 6.3 Earnings Losses Relative to Typical Nondisplaced Worker (Model (4.7)) and Relative to Workers in Displaced Workers' Former Firms (Model (4.24)): Workers in Growing or Modestly Declining Firms

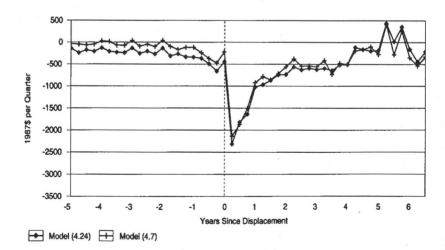

6.3   The Pattern of Earnings Losses by Industry

The findings in the two previous sections showed large earnings losses for workers separating from distressed firms, but smaller losses for other separators. One potential explanation for that difference is that distressed firms tend to be in the manufacturing sector, where workers earn substantial wage premiums as a result of unionization or rent sharing. Consequently, the sensitivity of earnings losses to the economic well-being of the firm might result from differences in industrial composition and not simply the firm's economic condition.

To explore this possibility, we limited our comparison of the losses suffered by manufacturing and nonmanufacturing workers to workers separating from distressed firms within those sectors. Figure 6.4 displays loss estimates corresponding to a version of specification (4.20) in which separate sets of displacement effects are estimated for manufacturing and nonmanufacturing workers and in which only mass layoff separators are included. For both groups the losses are relative to the earnings path that would have been expected based on the experiences of all nonseparators. As the figure shows, when analysis is limited to employees displaced from distressed firms, the earnings losses of nonmanufacturing and manufacturing workers are nearly the same. Therefore, the smaller earnings losses observed in chapter 5 for nonmanufacturing workers reflected differences between the shares of manufacturing and nonmanufacturing workers separating from distressed firms.[4]

To further explore the foregoing result, we examine the earnings losses for employees displaced from distressed firms in several broad sectors: nonmetals durable manufacturing firms, nondurable manufacturing firms, primary and fabricated metals firms, and firms in the trades, and the financial and services industries.[5] The main finding from these more disaggregated analyses is that the pattern of earnings losses is similar across broadly defined sectors of the economy. As shown by figure 6.5 and figure 6.6, we find similar earnings losses for workers displaced from distressed nondurable and nonmetals durable goods firms. Prior to separation, quarterly earnings of those workers decline modestly below their expected levels. Among the nonmetals durable goods workers that decline is not apparent until less than two years prior to displacement. After separation, earnings in both sectors fall sharply and remain $1,200 below their expected levels for most years after their discharges.

Figure 6.4   Earnings Losses for Manufacturing and Nonmanufacturing Workers: Workers Separating During Mass Layoffs

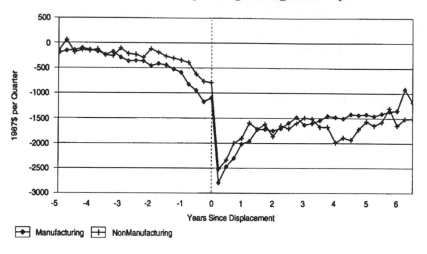

Figure 6.5   Earnings Losses in Nonmetals Durable Goods Industries: Workers Separating During Mass Layoffs

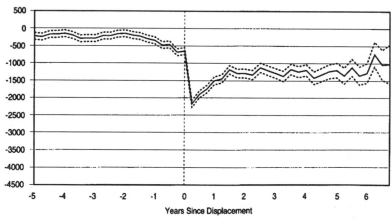

Figure 6.6   Earnings Losses in Nondurable Goods Industries: Workers Separating During Mass Layoffs

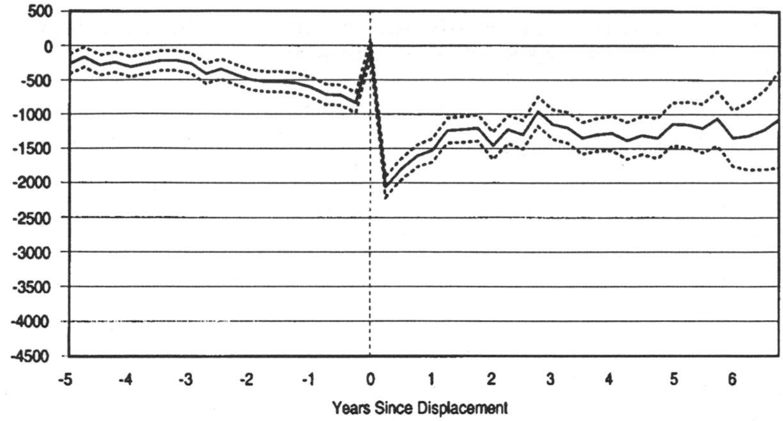

Estimate and 95% Confidence Interval Shown

Workers displaced from distressed firms in the trade, financial, and services sectors also experience substantial albeit smaller earnings losses. As shown by figure 6.7, prior to separation, those employees experience the smallest earnings losses, but after separation their earnings remain $1,000 below their expected levels. However, because these workers earned less than other workers before separation, their long-term losses are also approximately 25 percent of their predisplacement earnings. Therefore, except for some evidence of recovery after six years, workers displaced from distressed trades, and the financial and services firms experience losses similar to those experienced by displaced manufacturing workers.

The pattern of losses observed for workers displaced from the metals industries offers the most striking difference of any industry from the pattern observed in the previous figures. Displaced metals workers experienced earnings losses nearly double those of other displaced workers. As shown by figure 6.8, such workers experienced severe losses prior to their displacement,[6] even sharper losses immediately after separation, and four years later earn $2,500 less than their expected quarterly earnings. These losses represent approximately 35 percent of the predisplacement earnings of metal workers. Our analysis below shows that when we further disaggregate this sector, the losses for workers displaced from the primary metals industry substantially exceed the levels shown in the figure.

Figure 6.7   Earnings Losses in Trade and Services Industries: Workers Separating During Mass Layoffs

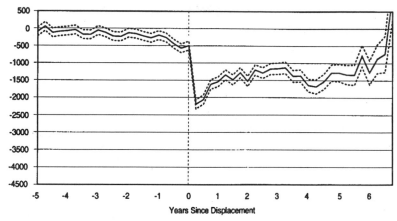

Years Since Displacement

Estimate and 95% Confidence Interval Shown

Figure 6.8   Earnings Losses in Metals Industries: Workers Separating During Mass Layoffs

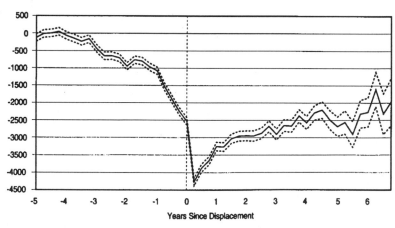

Years Since Displacement

Estimate and 95% Confidence Interval Shown

In order to further disaggregate our earnings loss estimates by industry, we must place some additional restrictions on the model (4.20). The difficulty we face in estimating such losses at, say, the 2-digit SIC industry level is that the numbers of displaced workers becomes too small relative to the number of parameters in the model. For example, if we wanted to estimate the pattern of losses for 20 separate industries, we would estimate 960 displacement effects corresponding to the 48 displacement coefficients for each industry. An even more practical problem associated with this approach is that the results are difficult to absorb even in a series of figures.

As discussed in chapter 4, we found that a more parsimonious version of the model given by (4.21) adequately summarizes the pattern of losses for each industry. According to this specification, rather than estimating a separate set of 48 displacement coefficients for each industry, we use three parameters to summarize how the pattern of losses for workers in a particular industry diverges from the pattern for the average displaced worker. These three components capture differences among groups' predisplacement earnings "dip," earnings "drop" after separation, and postdisplacement earnings "recovery." The "dip" parameter measures how much faster (or slower) a group's quarterly earnings declined during the 12 quarters before their job loss compared with the rate for the average displaced worker. The "drop" parameter measures a group's average postseparation earnings decline compared with the decline for the average displaced worker. Finally, the "recovery" parameter measures how much faster or slower a group's postdisplacement earnings recover after the sixth quarter following separation compared with the rate for the average displaced worker.

To illustrate that the foregoing restrictions on the model do not substantially alter our findings, we compared the pattern of losses for displaced manufacturing and nonmanufacturing workers given by the unrestricted model with those given by the more parsimonious specification. As shown by figure 6.9 and figure 6.10, both models generate nearly the same estimated earnings losses for both displaced manufacturing and nonmanufacturing workers.[7] Because the restricted model performs well, we use it to estimate differences in the pattern of losses for workers displaced from different industries.

Figure 6.9   Unrestricted Specification of Earnings Losses by Industrial Sector

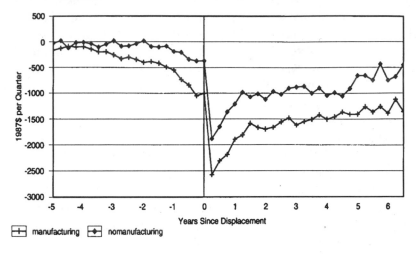

Figure 6.10   Parsimonious Specification of Earnings Losses by Industrial Sector: Workers in Surviving Firms

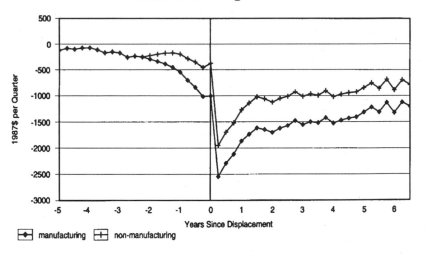

In the more highly disaggregated comparisons of earnings losses among industries presented below, we hold constant the effect of other worker characteristics on losses. For example, in the comparisons between earnings losses of displaced primary metals workers and financial workers, both groups, in effect, have the same distribution of sex, age, industry, regional characteristics, and local labor market conditions at the date of displacement. Therefore, the differences in losses between the two groups do not result from differences in the percentages of men and women in these industries. In the following two sections of this chapter, we show how the pattern of losses varies according to gender and age of workers, and labor market conditions at the time of their separations.

Loss estimates based on our parsimonious specification are shown in table 6.1.[8] Estimates in the column labeled "dip" show how a particular group's rate of quarterly earnings decline in the 13-quarter period immediately preceding separation differs from the average for all workers ($83 per quarter). Estimates in the column labeled "drop" show how a group's earnings losses in the period one to six quarters after displacement differs from that of the average worker ($2,179). Estimates in the column labeled "recovery" show how a group's rate of earnings recovery in the period seven or more quarters after displacement differs from that of the average worker ($15 per quarter). The column labeled "fifth-year loss dif" summarizes the effects of the drop and recovery coefficients for the size of the total loss in the fifth-year following displacement. Specifically, it gives the difference between a group's fifth-year loss and that of the average worker ($6,611). The last column, labeled "fifth-year loss," simply adds back the average loss to get the estimate of a group's total earnings losses during the fifth year after displacement.[9]

The results shown in table 6.1 indicate that although differences emerge in the earnings loss patterns for workers from different industries, generally displacement is associated with substantial long-term earnings losses. As shown by the last column of table 6.1, during the fifth year after displacement, losses exceed $4,500 for workers displaced from all but the financial and services sectors. To underscore the point that large earnings losses are experienced by workers outside the trade-sensitive, highly unionized durable goods industries, it is worth observing that the pattern of earnings losses for workers displaced from the wholesale and retail trade sector is more similar than any other to the pattern observed for the average displaced worker (summarized in the first row of the table). As shown by the first three

118

Table 6.1 Earnings Losses by Worker Characteristics: Parsimonious Specification

Group	Number	Dip	Drop	Recovery	Fifth-year loss dif.	Fifth-year loss
Overall	6,435	-83.3 (2.2)	2,179 (16)	15.4 (4.4)	—	-6,611 (150)
Sex						
Male	4,972	-3.4 (0.7)	-103 (7)	4.7 (0.9)	-177 (43)	-6,788 (157)
Female	1,463	11.6 (2.3)	350 (25)	-16.0 (3.2)	602 (145)	-6,009 (207)
Decade of birth						
1930s	2,599	-0.3 (1.4)	55 (16)	-10.1 (2.1)	-284 (94)	-6,896 (182)
1940s	2,584	3.6 (1.4)	-28 (15)	5.6 (2.0)	171 (88)	-6,440 (172)
1950s	1,252	-6.9 (2.4)	-58 (25)	9.4 (3.2)	238 (145)	-6,374 (203)
Industry						
Mining & construction	247	9.5 (5.8)	-387 (59)	-0.1 (7.8)	-1,549 (339)	-8,160 (369)
Nondurable manufacturing	1,206	18.3 (2.6)	338 (28)	-7.7 (3.7)	967 (160)	-5,644 (224)
Primary metals	1,354	-104.5 (2.7)	-1,476 (30)	40.5 (4.4)	-3,878 (191)	-10,489 (241)

Nonelectrical machinery	632	35.0 (3.5)	797 (39)	-27.4 (5.9)	1,817 (257)	-4,794 (306)
Electrical machinery	421	49.5 (4.3)	494 (47)	-2.7 (6.4)	1,842 (282)	-4,769 (322)
Transportation equipment	419	14.1 (4.4)	215 (48)	-15.5 6.6	85 (282)	-6,526 (324)
Other durable manufacturing	441	18.9 (4.2)	338 (43)	9.1 (5.7)	1,807 (242)	-4,804 (282)
Transportation, communication, and public utilities	348	5.5 (4.8)	66 (50)	-63.6 (7.1)	-2,916 (301)	-9,527 (333)
Wholesale and retail trade	545	20.0 (3.8)	126 (38)	4.8 (4.9)	745 (211)	-5,866 (251)
Finance, insurance, and real estate	183	115.7 (6.7)	947 (72)	24.3 (8.3)	5,004 (358)	-1,608 (387)
Professional, business and entertainment services	203	93.1 (6.4)	1,270 (64)	-26.2 (8.7)	3,769 (369)	-2,843 (394)
Firm size						
50-500	1,704	-16.1 (2.1)	-37 (22)	13.0 (2.9)	501 (124)	-6,110 (193)
501-2,000	1,497	13.9 (2.2)	214 (23)	-4.7 (3.1)	625 (135)	-5,986 (246)
2,001-5,000	1,381	27.2 (2.3)	480 (24)	-23.8 (3.5)	730 (149)	-5,881 (203)
Greater than 5,000	1,853	-16.7 (2.3)	-497 (25)	9.6 (3.6)	-1,510 (154)	-8,121 (224)

Group	Number	Dip	Drop	Recovery	Fifth-year loss dif.	Fifth-year loss
Local labor market						
Employment trend		38.8	743	18.1	2,069	
		(7.9)	(87)	(11.7)	(520)	
Employment deviation		517.7	3762	-40.9	-540	
		(64.4)	(645)	(94.1)	(408)	
Unemployment rate		11.9	-5,545	13.1	-2,153	
		(90.0)	(976)	(145.9)	(643)	

columns of table 6.1, losses for these workers depart modestly from the average pattern only in the predisplacement period, when their earnings decline at a slower rate than average. Nevertheless, during the fifth year following their job losses, losses for trades workers exceeded $5,800.

To be sure, job losses from heavily unionized industries are also associated with substantial earnings losses. We found the largest long-term losses for workers displaced from mining and construction, from primary metals, and from transportation, communications, and public utilities industries. These industries all have among the highest rates of unionization in the economy. Indeed, the pattern of losses for displaced workers in primary metals diverge substantially from the pattern depicted in figure 6.1. Prior to displacement, this group's earnings fall $104 per quarter faster than the average rate, and drop by $1,476 per quarter more than the average decline following separation. During the recovery period, however, their earnings grow $41 per quarter faster than the average rate of growth. However, despite that growth, during the fifth year after separation, earnings of these workers remain more than $10,000 below their expected levels. That loss exceeds 40 percent of their predisplacement wages.

The long-term losses are nearly as large for those displaced from the mining and construction and from the transportation, communications, and public utilities sectors. However, earnings loss patterns of these groups differ substantially from that observed for primary metals workers. During the predisplacement period, their earnings "dip" is similar to that of the average displaced worker, falling at rates only $9.5 and $5.5 per quarter slower than average. In the postseparation period, losses are much smaller for these groups than for primary metals workers. For example, the postseparation losses for displaced mining workers are $1,089 (-387 minus -1,476) less per quarter than those for primary metals workers. However, long-term losses remain large for mining and construction workers and for transportation, communications, and public utilities workers because their earnings grow more slowly during the recovery period than do those of displaced primary metals workers. As a result of this slow rate of growth, their earnings remain more than $8,000 below their expected levels in the fifth year following separation.

At the other extreme, workers displaced from the nonunion financial services sector experience much smaller losses than other groups. As indicated by table 6.1, earnings of financial services workers fall by $116 per quarter less than the average decline during the predisplacement period. This estimate implies that their preseparation earnings did not decline below expected levels. After they are displaced, earnings of these workers fall by $947 per quarter less than the average decline, and subsequently recover at a modestly faster rate than the rate for the average displaced worker. As a result, during the fifth year following their separations, earnings of displaced financial workers are only $1,600 below their expected levels. Although this estimate is relatively small, even in this strong industry, worker displacement is associated with modest long-term losses.

Another point apparent from table 6.1 is that workers generally recover very slowly from their earnings losses. Beginning with the seventh quarter following displacement, the average displaced worker's earnings loss recovers at a rate of only $15 per quarter. Only among displaced primary metals and financial sector workers is the rate of recovery substantially greater. At these rates of earnings recovery, only for younger workers would earnings converge with expected levels during their working lifetimes.

To further examine the pattern of earnings recovery among industries, we used our unrestricted model to compute the earnings losses for workers in each industry during the first, third, and fifth year following displacement. As shown by the first three columns of table 6.2, between the first and third years following job loss, earnings rise substantially relative to their expected levels. This rise results because workers are increasingly likely to be employed. However, beyond the third year, there is little evidence that earnings continue to recover. In only 11 of the 25 industries studied do the earnings loss estimates decline between the third and fifth year following separation.

The parsimonious version of the model also indicates that workers displaced from distressed financial services firms incur relatively small long-term losses. Their fifth-year losses amount to approximately 5 percent of their predisplacement earnings. One possible reason for these smaller losses is that displaced financial workers were able to find similar jobs because they had been displaced from a relatively strong industry. We observed in section 6.2 that the earnings of nondisplaced workers in distressed firms declined relative to other nondisplaced workers. That decline likely results because of the effects of adverse economic conditions on the firm. Likewise, there may be economic factors that similarly affect all nondisplaced workers within a given industry. For example, the displaced financial services workers may fare relatively well because earnings are growing more rapidly in their industry. If this is the case, their estimated earnings losses should increase if we use earnings histories of only nondisplaced financial services workers to compute their expected earnings. We explore the importance of this possibility by estimating earnings losses of displaced workers when using nondisplaced workers from the same industry as the comparison group.[10]

As shown by columns 4-6 of table 6.2, the magnitudes of our earnings loss estimates in several of the industries studied depend on which comparison group we use. As expected, long-term losses of displaced financial services workers rise significantly to nearly $7,000 per year. For most industries , however, estimates of long-term losses are either similar or smaller when using this alternative measure. Moreover, in three industries—apparel, leather, and primary metals— the estimated losses are substantially smaller than the estimated losses based on the comparison group of all nondisplaced workers. In the primary metals industry the long-term loss estimates decline by nearly one-half. The estimated losses are smaller in these industries because nondisplaced workers experience significantly slower earnings growth than nondisplaced workers elsewhere in the state. More generally, the modest gap between the two sets of estimates in table 6.2 indicates that the earnings growth between the groups of nondisplaced workers varies systematically among industries.

As we argued above, we prefer the set of estimates based on a comparison group corresponding to all nondisplaced workers, because these workers may be adversely affected by structural and policy changes. When we compare the earnings of displaced workers to those of their counterparts who remained employed in their former industries, we more than likely understate the losses associated with adverse structural changes. When assessing the effects of changes in public policy, however, we should consider the adverse consequences on displaced as well as nondisplaced workers. Nevertheless, the figures in table 6.2 make clear that, no matter which set of estimates one prefers, the disaggregated industry results indicate that when high-tenure workers leave distressed firms, their subsequent earnings usually remain substantially below their expected levels.

6.4 Earnings Losses by Demographic Characteristics

The foregoing finding also is consistent with our findings on how losses vary according to demographic characteristics of workers and labor market conditions at the time of their job loss. In this section, we employ the same parsimonious specification described above to show how, after controlling for the distribution of worker characteristics, earnings losses vary only slightly according to gender and age.

As shown by table 6.1, we find similar earnings loss patterns among male and female displaced workers. However, modest differences do exist, as men's earnings fall by more prior to displacement and are lower in the period immediately after their job losses. Further, during the recovery period, men's earnings grow at a faster rate than do women's earnings. Despite these differences between men's and women's earnings loss patterns, both groups experience substantial long-term earnings losses. In the fifth year following job loss, men's earnings are $6,560 below their expected levels, whereas women's losses are nearly as large at $5,997. Moreover, because women's predisplacement earnings were only 60 percent those of men, the percentage earnings losses are actually larger for women. Indeed, because of the differences in their respective rates of recovery, in subsequent years the absolute difference between men's and women's long-term losses is likely to narrow while the percentage difference is likely to widen.

The earnings loss pattern also is similar among displaced workers from different age groups. Although younger workers experience larger earnings declines both prior to and at the time of separation and experience faster recovery rates, their earnings losses are nearly the same as they are for older workers during the fifth year following separation. However, the "recovery" coefficients suggest that the gap between the losses of younger and older workers should grow modestly at a rate of $19 per quarter. That difference suggests that younger workers are acquiring somewhat more human capital in their new careers than are their older counterparts. For this reason, if the difference in recovery rates persists, the sum of the discounted quarterly earnings losses during these workers' lifetimes will be larger for older workers, even though for the period covered by our sample, the discounted losses do not depend much on age. However, overall our findings indicate that displacement is extremely costly, even for high-tenure younger workers.

6.5 Earnings Losses and Local Labor Market Conditions

We find more substantial differences in earnings loss patterns when we compare displaced workers in different regions of Pennsylvania. Workers separating from distressed firms in the state's western section experience the largest losses, both as a result of larger predisplacement earnings declines and larger earnings drops in the period immediately following separation. By contrast, workers in the state's eastern section have much smaller predisplacement earnings declines, and their earnings drop by less after separation. However, because of slower postseparation rates of recovery, there were only modest differences in the losses incurred by workers in the long term in most parts of the state.

Displaced workers from southeastern Pennsylvania, especially those displaced from distressed firms in the Philadelphia SMSA, do fare substantially better than their counterparts elsewhere in the state. Their earnings decline by less prior to displacement, drop by less when they lose their jobs, and rise more rapidly during the recovery period than the earnings of displaced workers in other regions of the state. In the fifth year following separation, their earnings losses are more than $2,900 less than those of their counterparts in the region encompassing the state's other large metropolitan area—Pittsburgh.

Because the foregoing results take into account differences in the distribution of industries among regions, differences in industrial composition cannot account for the smaller losses observed in Philadelphia. A more compelling explanation for the differences in earnings losses is the widely differing labor market conditions that prevailed in Pennsylvania during the 1980s. The economic conditions in western Pennsylvania are substantially worse than those in the eastern part of the state. Although Pittsburgh, in the state's western section, and Philadelphia, in the state's eastern section, experience similar unemployment rates during the late 1970s, their rates during the 1980s diverge dramatically. Only in the second half of the decade do the rates approach each other. Movements of employment levels in these areas also indicate substantial differences in their labor market conditions. During the 1980s, employment levels in Pittsburgh remained 5 percent below their late 1970s average, while those in Philadelphia grew. The reason for the two regions' sharply different rates of employment growth is the much larger decline in manufacturing employment in Pittsburgh than in Philadelphia.

One reason why these regional labor market conditions differ is that the 1982 recession hit harder in some regions than in others. Because the severity of the recession varied among regions, the earnings loss pattern varied as well. Another reason has less to do with cyclical conditions and more to do with long-term economic conditions in the region. Some areas, such as Johnstown, have been depressed for many years, while at the same time other areas, such as Lancaster, have been prosperous. This view suggests that we should think of the effects of local labor market conditions on earnings losses as having two components. First, the cyclical component measures the effects of having been displaced during a strong or weak phase of the business cycle. And second, the secular component measures the effects of long-term conditions in the region. In our framework, the secular component is captured by the rate of growth in nonagricultural employment between 1976 and 1987. The cyclical component is captured by local unemployment rates and the deviations of local employment from its trend.

To make our results easier to interpret, the estimates in the last three rows of table 6.1 present the differences in earnings losses corresponding roughly to the best and worst economic conditions observed in Pennsylvania. The range of employment growth rates is approximately 1 percent per quarter; and the range of the unemployment rates and employment deviations from trend is approximately 10 percentage points. For example, the 5,545 figure in table 6.1 corresponding to the "drop" coefficient for the local unemployment rate suggests that being displaced in a locale where the unemployment rate is 10 percentage points above the "natural" rate raises the loss after separation by an enormous 5,545 per quarter more than the average loss. If the local unemployment rate were only 1 percentage point above its "natural" level, the loss per quarter would be $554 larger than average. As other studies have found, this result indicates that cyclical conditions have a substantial effect on short-term earnings losses of displaced workers.

In the long term, the results in table 6.1 indicate that cyclical conditions at the time of worker displacement continue to have a significant, although smaller, effect on earnings losses. The estimates for unemployment rates and employment deviations from trend indicate that the former variable captures the effect of cyclical conditions on the magnitude of the earnings "drop" at the time of worker displacement, but how these conditions affect the pattern of losses leading up to separation and the recovery afterwards is better captured by the latter variable. Together, the two variables indicate that being displaced during the worst as opposed to the best cyclical conditions raises losses during the fifth year following separation by -$1,613 (or -$2,153 minus -$540). Although this estimate is large, it also corresponds to unusually poor cyclical conditions. A more common event than the one depicted in the table would be for a worker to be displaced during a period when the unemployment rate was, say, 4 percentage points above the "natural" rate. In this instance, our results suggest that during the fifth year after separation, the losses of these workers were only $645 (0.4 times $1,613) larger than average. Therefore, we conclude that cyclical conditions at the time of job loss have long-lasting effects on earnings, but the effects are small compared to overall losses.

A region's secular economic conditions also have long-lasting and relatively modest effects on earnings losses. During the quarter prior to their job loss, workers displaced in the weakest local economies have earnings losses $500 (13 times 38.8) larger than those displaced in the strongest local economies. This gap widens to approximately $750 per quarter after displacement. Although there are faster rates of recovery in weaker labor markets, the gap remains at approximately $500 per quarter or $2,000 annually during the fifth year following job loss. Although these effects of local labor conditions are significant, it is important to recognize that according to our find-

Table 6.2 Annual Earnings Losses by Years Since Displacement for Workers Separating from Firms in Manufacturing

	Separations During Mass Layoffs			Comparisons from Separators' Industries		
	1 year	3 years	5 years	1 year	3 years	5 years
Panel A: 2-Digit Manufacturing Industries						
Food products	$-8,545	$-5,709	$-5,285	$-8,245	$-5,353	$-5,003
Tobacco	-5,236	-3,418	-4,803	-4,002	-2,028	-3,310
Textile mill	-6,428	-3,989	-4,770	-4,914	-2,227	-2,244
Apparel	-6,660	-4,931	-6,474	-4,447	-2,303	-3,285
Wood products	-8,686	-4,586	-1,914	-6,757	-2,464	373
Furniture and fixtures	-4,199	-1,941	-2,546	-3,430	-1,038	-1,578
Paper and pulp	-,5516	-,3409	-4,283	-6,590	-4,679	-6,075
Printing and publishing	-9,305	-6,539	-6,240	-9,368	-6,866	-7,210
Chemicals	-4995	-2,527	-2,756	-6,399	-4,116	-4,850
Petroleum and coal products	-6,075	-1,451	-2,154	-9,882	-5,808	-3,359
Rubber	-8,285	-5,520	-5,223	-8,245	-5,538	-5,518
Leather	-7,929	-5,875	-6,844	-4,542	-1,817	-1,765
Stone, glass, clay, concrete	-8,261	-5,771	-5,964	-8,283	-5,770	-6,095
Primary metals	-17,365	-13,695	-11,790	-14,133	-9,498	-6,050
Fabricated metals	-7,194	-4,717	-4,932	-6,357	-3,762	-3,946
Nonelectrical machinery	-5,714	-3,716	-4,781	-4,003	-1,748	-2,532
Electrical machinery	-8,555	-5,759	-5,407	-10,235	-6,277	-6,129
Transportation equipment	-7,991	-5,819	-6,576	-7,758	-5,027	-6,145
Professional equipment	-7,824	-5,312	-5,465	-7,852	-4,780	-4,120

Panel B: 1-Digit Nonmanufacturing Industries

Other goods	11,553	-8,931	-8,889	-9,998	-7,045	-6,586
Transportation, communications, public utilities	-9,078	-7,559	-9,478	-10,493	-9,263	-11,870
Wholesale, retail trade	-8,827	-6,106	-5,888	-7,872	-4,948	-4,541
Financial, insurance, real estate	-4,606	-1,693	-1,133	-7,830	-5,799	-6,981
Business and personal services	-5,783	-3,090	-2,919	-5,515	-2,883	-2,998
Professional services	-4,696	-2,640	-3,602	-3,600	-1,223	-1,789

NOTE: Earnings losses are given for 1, 3, and 5 years following workers separation.

ings, job loss is associated with substantial earnings losses even in the strongest of labor markets.

Besides their direct effect on the magnitude of displaced worker earnings losses, local labor market conditions also affect incentives for workers to move to areas where they face better prospects. The varying economic conditions among regions suggests that workers do face such incentives. Indeed, one concern raised in chapter 3 when we described our data was that our estimates may overstate losses because the more successful displaced workers moved out of state in pursuit of better prospects. Although our data do not permit us to directly explore that possibility, we can examine how losses vary depending on whether workers' new firms were located in different regions within Pennsylvania.

Our data indicate that by 1986, approximately one-third of the displaced workers in our mass layoff sample were employed in firms located in SMSAs (or in a different county for persons previously employed in firms located outside SMSAs) that were different from the SMSA of their 1979 employer. This measure exaggerates the amount of migration, because larger firms may have plants located in several regions, but in our data firm location does not vary by plant. Despite this shortcoming associated with our measure of mobility, it does behave like more conventional measures in that younger workers and men are more likely to have moved.

With this caveat in mind, we find that, on average, movers suffer long-term losses $400 per quarter larger than those who stayed in their regions. These findings suggest that workers likely to incur larger losses are more likely to move. But moving does not reduce their losses even to the level of otherwise similar persons who stayed in their area. In addition, these findings suggest that if we had data on persons who moved out-of-state, the overall earnings loss estimates might be larger, not smaller, than those reported in this chapter.

6.6 Earnings Losses and Industry of New Job

In previous sections, we showed that regardless of their former firms' industry, their demographic characteristics, or the labor market conditions at the time of their separation, high-tenure workers usually incur substantial earnings losses when they are displaced from distressed firms. Another potential determinant of displaced worker earnings losses is the industry of their new jobs. For example, workers displaced from distressed manufacturing firms may fare better if they find new jobs in the manufacturing as opposed to the nonmanufacturing sector. One reason for such a relationship is that some worker skills may be specific to a particular sector, industry, or firm. When displaced workers find new jobs that are similar to their old jobs, they are able to continue to use those specialized skills. As a result, their earnings losses should be relatively small. In contrast, if the new jobs of displaced workers are sufficiently different from their old jobs, those specialized skills will go unused, with larger earnings losses the likely result.

In keeping with this study's interest in the long-term impacts of displacement, we want to assess the relationship between earnings losses and the industry of workers' new jobs several years following their separations. For workers displaced in 1985 and 1986 such an assessment is impossible because we have only a few quarters of postseparation data. Accordingly, we examined the relationship between earnings losses and industry of the new job for workers displaced from distressed firms between 1980 and 1983. The industry of the new job was the workers' primary employer in 1986.

As shown by figure 6.11, earnings losses of manufacturing workers depend crucially on whether their new jobs were in the same sector as their old jobs. When displaced manufacturing workers found new jobs in the manufacturing sector, their earnings losses five years after separation averaged approximately $1,000 per quarter. That loss represents about 20 percent of their expected earnings. In contrast, when their new jobs were in the nonmanufacturing sector, their quarterly earnings losses rose to approximately $2,000 per quarter. That loss represents nearly 40 percent of their expected earnings. These findings underscore the importance to displaced manufacturing workers of finding new jobs in their old sector.

Turning to displaced workers from the nonmanufacturing sector, we find in figure 6.12 that these workers also incurred substantial losses no matter in which sector they end up. For those workers who remained in the nonmanufacturing sector, their earnings losses were similar to the losses for manufacturing workers who remained in their old sector. Once again, the earnings losses are smaller when displaced workers' new jobs were in the same sector as their old jobs. On average, those displaced nonmanufacturing workers who switched sectors experienced larger earnings losses. But there are two reasons that the evidence on this relationship is less conclusive for nonmanufacturing workers: First, relatively few displaced nonmanufacturing workers found jobs in the manufacturing sector. That fact accounts, in part, for larger variability in the earnings loss estimates for workers who switched sectors. Second, in some years the earnings losses of the sector stayers and sector switchers were similar.

Figure 6.11 Manufacturing Workers' Earnings Losses by Sector of Postdisplacement Job

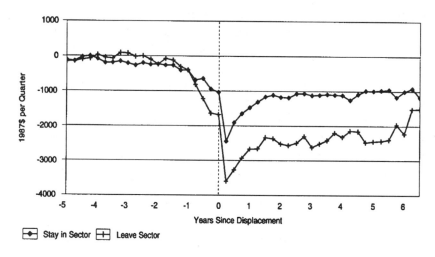

The evidence presented in figure 6.11 and figure 6.12 indicates that the earnings losses of displaced workers, would be reduced if they found new jobs in their old sectors. To pursue this point further, we examined the earnings losses among two groups of workers whose new jobs were in their old sectors. The first group found a new job in the same 4-digit SIC industry as their old job. The second group found a new job in the same sector but in a different 4-digit industry. Underlying this characterization of the new jobs is the assumption that when they are in the same 4-digit SIC industry as the old jobs they are more likely to require skills similar to those used in the former positions. Accordingly, the earnings losses for those workers should, on average, be less than for workers whose new jobs are in different industries from their former jobs.

Figure 6.12 Nonmanufacturing Workers' Earnings Losses by Sector of Postdisplacement Job

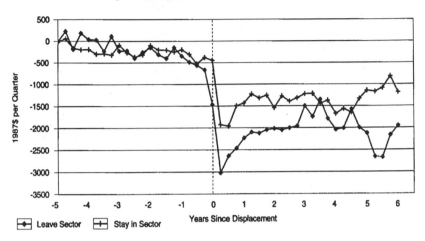

Surprisingly, we find that even when the new jobs are in the same 4-digit SIC industry as the old jobs, earnings losses of displaced workers are substantial. As shown in Panel A of table 6.3, 24 quarters after their separations, earnings of displaced manufacturing workers are 20 percent below expected levels when their new jobs are in the same 4-digit industry as their old jobs. Further, those losses are similar to those experienced by workers who find less similar jobs in the manufacturing sector. That percentage loss is 18 percent for workers who remain in the manufacturing sector but are employed in a different 4-digit SIC industry. By comparison, the losses jump to 38 percent for workers whose new jobs are in the nonmanufacturing sector.

Table 6.3 Earnings Losses by Sector of New Jobs

Quarters since separation	New job in same sector		New job in other sector
	Same 4-digit SIC	Different 4-digit SIC	
Panel A: Displaced Manufacturing Workers			
-8	$-379	$-117	$-237
	(82)	(67)	(73)
	[-7]	[-2]	[-4]
12	-1,044	-1,117	-2,616
	(82)	(67)	(73)
	[-19]	[-21]	[-44]
24	-1,103	-958	-2,221
	(197)	(137)	(150)
	[-20]	[-18]	[-38]
Panel B: Displaced Nonmanufacturing Workers			
-8	$-229	$-26	$-151
	(132)	(128)	(231)
	[-18]	[0]	[-3]
12	-1,129	-1,305	-1,498
	(132)	(128)	(231)
	[-18]	[-23]	[-26]
24	-1,103	-1,276	-1,949
	(315)	(241)	(476)
	[-18]	[-22]	[-33]

The findings for displaced nonmanufacturing workers are similar to those for their manufacturing counterparts. When displaced nonmanufacturing workers find new jobs in the same 4-digit industry, their long-term earnings losses amount to 18 percent. That percentage rises to 22 percent when their new jobs are in a new 4-digit industry but still in the nonmanufacturing sector. By comparison, losses rise to 34 percent for those who find new jobs in the manufacturing sector. But, because so few displaced nonmanufacturing workers move to the manufacturing sector, this rise in losses is not statistically significant. However, we find no evidence that displaced nonmanufacturing workers have smaller losses if they find new jobs in the manufacturing sector.

Most notably, the two sets of results in table 6.3 for manufacturing and nonmanufacturing workers indicate that even when displaced

Most notably, the two sets of results in table 6.3 for manufacturing and nonmanufacturing workers indicate that even when displaced workers find new jobs in their former industry, they still incur long-term losses of between 15 and 20 percent. In light of our earlier finding that displaced workers in most industries suffer substantial earnings losses, these findings suggest that much of their earnings losses result from factors specific to their old firms. These specific factors might include specific human capital, the value of the employer and employee "match," or the workings of internal labor markets.

6.7 Conclusions

This chapter emphasized the link between earnings losses of displaced workers and the economic health of their former firms. In general, when high-tenure workers separated from their firms between 1980 and 1986, their earnings declined significantly. For those separating from distressed firms, however, the declines were substantial and persisted at least for six years. For other separators, the earnings losses were smaller, and indeed the earnings of groups actually returned to their expected levels after several years.

Among workers separating from distressed firms, the following points are clear. First, about one-fifth of their earnings loss would have occurred even had they not been displaced. In distressed firms, the earnings of nondisplaced workers decline relative to other nondisplaced workers. Second, high-tenure workers are vulnerable to displacement no matter which sector they work in, and regardless of their gender or age and of the prevailing local labor market conditions at the time of their displacements. Finally, the evidence on the relationship between earnings losses of displaced workers and the industry of their new jobs indicates that a substantial portion of those losses results from the loss of some attribute of the employment relationship. In the next chapter we will consider some of the policy implications of these findings.

136   Earnings Losses and Mass Layoffs

NOTES

1. For convenience, we sometimes refer to workers from such distressed firms as "mass lay-off" workers even though the category includes workers whose firms shut down completely.

2. If the preseparation earnings losses result from errors in dating those separations, the findings in figure 6.1 suggests that those dating errors are more likely when employees separate from firms experiencing large workforce reductions. Because we do not know of any *a priori* reason for why this result should be the case, we believe that figure 6.1 provides additional evidence against the dating hypothesis described in chapter 3.

3. For example, we have no evidence that many workers in our sample receive piece rates. Earnings of such workers would decline as a result of declining productivity.

4. In results not shown here we find that losses of manufacturing and nonmanufacturing workers were also nearly the same (and much smaller than shown in figure 6.4) when the analysis is limited to nonmass layoff separators.

5. Again, the estimates shown in figures 6.5 through 6.8 are of the δ_{jt} parameters in model (4.20). In particular, these estimates allow for common estimates of the quarter (time) and age effects.

6. As in note 1 above, the large predisplacement earnings for displaced metals workers appears to work against the dating hypothesis described in chapter 3. According to this hypothesis, the extremely large preseparation losses depicted in figure 6.8 suggest that dating errors occur more often for workers displaced from metals firms than for workers displaced from other manufacturing firms.

7. The estimates shown in figure 6.9 and figure 6.10 were obtained using the full sample of high attachment separators who in 1979 were in firms that survived to the end of the sample period. This change in samples explains the differences between these figures and figure 6.4, which was obtained using all workers in the mass layoff sample including workers separating from firms that closed.

8. In this section we discuss only the results in the industry panel of table 6.1. The other results in the table are discussed in sections 6.4 and 6.5.

9. See chapter 4 for discussion of the parsimonious specification.

10. Operationally, as in equation (4.23), we computed the estimates for the last three columns of table 6.1 by adding industry-specific time trends to the econometric model.

7
Conclusions and
Policy Considerations

The central finding of this study is that high-tenure workers suffer large losses when they are displaced as part of plant closings or mass layoffs. When these workers separate from distressed firms, their earnings fall dramatically below the levels that we otherwise would expect. During the year following their separations, their losses are especially great. For the period covered by this study, 1980 to 1986, these losses averaged about $9,000 or 40 percent of predisplacement earnings. Although these losses decline somewhat with time, they did not disappear. Even during the fifth year after job separation, their losses averaged approximately $6,500 or 25 percent of former earnings. As a result, the average present discounted value of earnings losses during the period from three years before to six years after separation amounts to approximately $50,000. If, as seems likely, earnings losses remained at about $6,000 per year until retirement (at age 65), the present value of losses rose to approximately $80,000. Clearly, displacement is a major setback for experienced workers.

We also find that displacement affects a great many experienced workers. The 6,435 workers in our 5 percent sample suggest that 135,000 high-tenure workers left distressed firms in Pennsylvania between 1980 and 1986. Moreover, if the experience of Pennsylvania is representative of the nation as a whole, then during this period approximately 2.6 million such U.S. workers were displaced from distressed firms. In fact, our tabulations of the Displaced Workers Surveys covering the years 1979 to 1985 also suggest that 2.6 million prime-age American workers with six or more years of tenure were displaced during that nearly identical seven-year period. These figures demonstrate that even among experienced workers, job loss is a significant threat.

Together, these two findings—that displacement is a major financial setback and that it threatens many high-tenure workers—substantiate workers' concerns about the possibility and consequences of job loss. Indeed, our findings imply that the economic well-being of their firms is an important determinant of workers' own labor market success. Two equally talented and hard-working individuals will not necessarily do equally well in the labor market if one of them works for a firm that is unsuccessful. Rather, if the unsuccessful firm is forced to lay off one of these workers, our findings suggest that he or she is likely to earn significantly less than the other worker for many years. The importance of job loss explains the concerns of labor unions and sympathetic policymakers about policies such as trade liberalization or environmental protection that may lead to increased displacement.

Our results explain why workers should be concerned about displacement. They do not, however, necessarily imply that policymakers should attempt to allay those concerns by providing displaced workers with assistance generous enough to fully compensate for their losses. The extent to which policymakers should create programs to assist displaced workers or compensate them for their losses is fundamentally a political question that depends on judgments beyond the scope of this monograph. Nevertheless, our study has several implications about the efficacy of existing and alternative programs. To facilitate that discussion, we briefly recount the reasons policymakers and others have given for assisting displaced workers. These reasons fall into four categories: (1) it is simply the fair thing to do; (2) it is desirable on income distribution grounds; (3) it corrects a market failure that occurs because of a missing insurance market; and (4) it promotes efficiency by facilitating change that would otherwise be politically impossible. We briefly comment on each of these views below.

Perhaps the most commonly cited reason for assisting displaced workers is simple fairness. Some policymakers take the view that workers who have maintained stable employment relationships over a number of years have "played by the rules" and therefore are entitled to a secure economic future. Accordingly, they argue it is simply unfair to allow workers to suffer large losses when events beyond their control put them out of work. This unfairness seems especially great to many because these same events (for example, technological progress, freer trade, or a healthier, more attractive environment) usually benefit the rest of society. Because it is based on a notion of fairness, there is little we can say analytically about this argument beyond that it seems most compelling when the displacement is caused by a change in government policy. For example, when the government acts to protect an endangered species and thereby causes workers to lose valuable employment relationships, the government has, in a sense, seized the workers' property and thus owes them compensation.

Those concerned about the increasing extent of income inequality and the "erosion of the middle class" also have advocated compensation for displaced workers. Given such concerns, the appeal of assisting displaced workers is easy to understand. Before their job losses, the workers we studied were solidly middle class, with average incomes somewhat above the median, while after their setbacks many had incomes low enough to threaten their middle-class status. On average, providing compensation to displaced workers probably does contribute to greater income equality. However, as a tool for achieving this end, it is a very blunt instrument. Workers who have held a job for more than a decade are not likely to be among society's neediest even after being displaced. Indeed, we find, as have other studies, that many displaced workers have earnings above the median even after their displacements (Kosters 1986).

Compensating displaced workers also might be justified as the response to a market failure caused by the inability of workers to insure fully against the risk of displacement. For a number of reasons private insurers probably cannot profitably provide such insurance. For instance, workers are likely to know much more than any insurer about the likelihood that a mass layoff or plant closing will lead to job loss. Thus private insurers would attract mostly high-risk workers and likely find such a business unprofitable. Unfortunately, without the ability to insure against displacement, workers will, to an extent greater than socially desirable, avoid jobs with above-average layoff risk. Of course, firms may attempt to lure workers into such jobs by paying them higher wages (as a form of compensating differential). But, the necessity of paying higher wages because of the unavailability of insurance will also cause firms to hire fewer workers than is socially desirable. Therefore, these wage premiums only partially alleviate the inefficiency caused by this missing market. We know of no empirical evidence on the magnitude of this efficiency loss, but, in principle, governmentally provided insurance in the form of a guarantee of compensation in the event of displacement could enhance efficiency by allowing workers to take jobs with less certain outcomes without at the same time unduly increasing labor costs of firms.

A final argument for assisting displaced workers is that unless they provide this assistance, policymakers may be unable to enact beneficial public policies. History suggests that workers who would be adversely affected by a proposed policy change may successfully lobby against that change even if, on net, it would benefit society. Likewise, groups adversely affected by technological progress or taste shifts may seek governmental regulations that block those changes. Of course, when a change brings society net benefits, then those who gain could, in principle, compensate those who lose and still be better off themselves. This observation underlies economists' support for trade liberalization and many other "free market" policies. However, in the absence of a mechanism for actually carrying out such compensation, this reasoning is less compelling. Moreover, regardless of the merits of economists' arguments, policies with the greatest net benefit to society might not be adopted if the minority who would lose have more political might than the majority who would gain. The actual alternative to providing generous assistance to those adversely affected by technological or policy changes may be accepting trade restrictions, subsidization of inefficient firms, and a less healthy environment.

In the past these rationales have motivated policymakers to design several programs to assist displaced workers. Some of these programs also are aimed at the general population of unemployed persons. Other programs are aimed specifically at displaced workers. The unemployment insurance (UI) system provides the most basic form of assistance to a broad class of unemployed job losers. The Trade Adjustment Assistance (TAA) program extends the duration of UI payments (and provides retraining vouchers) to a narrower population of unemployed persons whose job loss the Secretary of Labor has certified resulted from import competition.

In addition, policymakers have supplemented these income replacement programs with programs that provide employment and training services. At the broadest level of targeting, each state operates an Employment Service (ES) as a labor exchange to help the unemployed find work. A much more comprehensive set of services is available to workers covered by the Economic Dislocation and Worker Adjustment Assistance Act (EDWAA). These services include more extensive job search assistance, counseling, and formal training. In addition, until recently, financial assistance for postsecondary education was also available to displaced workers under a special provision of the Pell Grant program. Finally, the requirement that employers give advance notice before laying off large numbers of workers also is designed to facilitate the job search of those who subsequently are displaced. These programs, discussed at greater length below, are evidence of policymakers' desire to provide assistance to displaced workers.

Unfortunately, our results on the magnitude and temporal pattern of displaced worker earnings losses imply that the existing array of programs does not, and probably cannot, eliminate more than a small fraction of such losses. This conclusion stems from our finding that workers suffer the majority of their losses in the form of reduced earnings after they find new jobs. The implication of this finding is that programs such as UI and TAA, which provide cash payments to workers only while they are unemployed, can compensate them only for a small portion of their losses. In addition, previous research on the impacts of job search assistance and retraining programs provides little cause for optimism that such programs can go very far towards reducing the sizable losses found in this study.

In what follows, we suggest some changes to the existing set of programs, but the failure of existing programs to substantially reduce earnings losses largely reflects real difficulties inherent in their design. No matter how committed policymakers are to assisting those who bear the costs of change, they may simply be unable to do so within the framework of existing programs. Compensating displaced workers for a substantially larger fraction of their losses likely requires an alternative, and more costly, approach in which income support extends beyond the period workers are unemployed.

The remainder of this chapter proceeds as follows. In section 7.1 we present a more detailed summary of our results, along with some general implications for policies designed to assist displaced workers. In section 7.2 we discuss in greater detail the relevance of our findings for the existing array of government programs in this area. In section 7.3 we offer some more speculative thoughts on how a wage subsidy program might be designed to more fully compensate displaced workers. Finally, section 7.4 contains some brief conclusions.

7.1 Summary of Findings

This section summarizes our monograph's most important empirical findings and notes their general implications for public policy. We begin by decomposing the average worker's earnings losses into several distinct components. This decomposition serves a number of purposes. First, it shows that the existing array of programs cannot begin to compensate displaced workers for their full losses. Second, it illustrates the complications that would necessarily entail a hypothetical program designed to provide full or nearly full compensation to displaced workers. Finally, it makes clear the virtues of our data and the analysis they allow relative to other research designs. After discussing this decomposition, we go on to briefly indicate how the effects of displacement vary among workers. These results show which earnings losses might merit the special attention of policymakers. They also provide some hints about the importance of the different theoretical rationales discussed in chapter 1 for why earnings losses might occur.

Figure 7.1, which is a modified version of figure 4.1, illustrates the decomposition of the average displaced worker's losses that we find useful for discussing policies towards the displaced. The bottom line in the figure depicts the earnings path of that worker while the top line depicts the earnings path of an otherwise identical nondisplaced worker. The figure indicates two dates: (1) the date when the worker separates from his or her old employer, and (2) the date when that worker establishes a stable employment relationship with a new employer. Also indicated in the figure are the worker's earnings on the separation date. The displaced worker's losses for any particular quarter are given by the vertical distance between the two earnings paths. Several figures in chapters 5 and 6 plot estimates of these losses for various categories of workers. For workers separating amidst mass layoffs or plant closings, those figures revealed significant losses as early as three years prior to separation. Losses gradually rose to about $1,100 per quarter at the date of separation, before

increasing sharply to nearly $3,000 per quarter immediately after sep-
aration. Subsequently, earnings losses declined steadily for about six
quarters and then declined only gradually to a level around $1,500 per
quarter six years after displacement. Our estimate of the cumulative
loss corresponds to the (properly discounted) area between the lines
in figure 7.1.

The decomposition depicted in figure 7.1 helps us to better understand the importance of the following issues: (1) the relative importance of earnings losses due to unemployment following job
separation and losses due to lower earnings after reemployment; (2)
the importance of accounting for the dip in earnings that precedes
final job separation; (3) the loss resulting from lost earnings growth;
and (4) the portion of the loss due to our choice of a comparison
group of nondisplaced workers.

**Figure 7.1 Stylized Earnings Histories of Displaced Worker and Similar
Nondisplaced Worker**

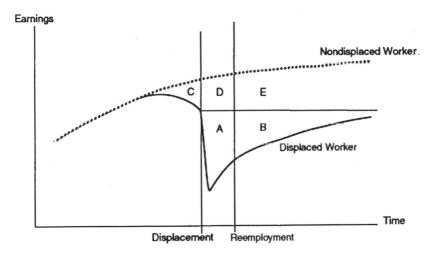

It is sometimes assumed that the costs of displacement are synony-
mous with earnings losses due to unemployment.[1] Our results show
that this is far from the case. While the workers whose job losses we
studied varied greatly in the speed with which they found new work,
almost all of them had found stable employment by six quarters after

their separations. Average earnings losses during this transition period, which correspond to the sum of areas A and D in figure 7.1, were nearly $13,000. Only a portion of these losses (area D) is attributable to unemployment. But, even if unemployment was responsible for all of the losses during this period, it would still only account for about 16 percent of workers' cumulative earnings losses.

An obvious but important implication of this finding is that programs such as UI and TAA that provide income to workers only while they are unemployed cannot in their present forms come close to compensating displaced workers for their full losses. Of course, if the amount of UI payments and their maximum duration were significantly increased, workers would likely stay unemployed longer, increasing compensation from these programs. But, because it would delay reemployment, such a policy could be costly to the economy and might not increase the fraction of earnings losses covered.

Our results show that permanently lower quarterly earnings after reemployment account for the vast majority of earnings losses. Our estimate of the present discounted value of the losses occurring seven or more quarters after separation, which corresponds to the sum of areas B and E in figure 7.1, is approximately $58,000 or 72 percent of the cumulative losses. The fact that most of the earnings losses occur after the displaced return to work implies that if policymakers want to compensate for more of earnings losses, they need to design programs that raise workers' incomes after they find new employment. In principle, policymakers could achieve this objective by funding training programs that upgrade skills or job search assistance programs that better match workers' existing skills with the needs of employers. However, in the next section we note that the previous research on the impact of these programs provides little reason for optimism about the ability of policymakers to compensate for the sizable losses reported in this monograph. Later in this chapter, we outline a program that would raise the post-reemployment income of displaced workers by providing them with earnings or income subsidies.

Our finding that workers begin to experience earnings losses up to three years before separating from their employers has important implications for the measurement of overall earnings losses. First, the present value of the losses that occur before separation, corresponding to area C in figure 7.1, is far from negligible, amounting to approximately $9,000 or 12 percent of cumulative losses. Our results on the receipt of UI payments attribute about half of these losses to lost earnings while on temporary layoff. Thus, in contrast to the losses incurred after workers secure new employment, a significant fraction of the losses suffered before separation are offset by conventional UI benefits.[2]

Recognizing the importance of the preseparation earnings dip also allows us to avoid substantially underestimating earnings losses during the period after separation. As we noted in chapter 2, researchers using the Displaced Workers Surveys, which report only one preseparation observation on wages, may have done just that. If we used the earnings levels immediately prior to separation as a basis for calculating quarterly losses, our estimate of the total losses during the transition period following job loss (region A in figure 7.1) would decline to $7,000 and our estimate of the losses following reemployment (region B in figure 7.1) would decline to $12,000. Combined, these losses amount to $19,000 or less than 25 percent of what we report as the true losses. Therefore, failure to recognize the existence of the preseparation earnings dip could potentially lead to a very substantial underestimate of the total losses. One practical implication of these preseparation earnings losses is that programs designed to compensate workers for a substantial fraction of their losses may need to make assistance levels dependent on worker earnings during a period beginning several years prior to displacement.

The upper boundaries of regions C, D, and E in figure 7.1 depend on the rate of earnings growth in the absence of displacement. In other words, our measure of losses recognizes that lost earnings growth is just as injurious to displaced workers as actual earnings declines. Thus research designs that fail to consider the expected path of earnings in the absence of displacement underestimate losses if, in the absence of displacement, earnings would have grown. Again, we note in chapter 2 that studies using the Displaced Workers Surveys, which lack a comparison group of nondisplaced workers, suffer from this shortcoming. Although the period we studied was not one of particularly rapid, economywide earnings growth, our results in chapter 3 suggest that had we not taken lost earnings growth into consideration, our average loss estimates would be about 20 percent less. Moreover, earnings growth rates vary substantially by age, being most rapid for younger workers. As a result, accounting for lost earnings growth substantially raised our estimates of the relative losses of younger workers.

The importance of lost earnings growth to our estimates of total losses implies that a hypothetical program providing full compensation to displaced workers would have to be quite complex. Payments would need to depend on a worker's age and sex (raising legal issues of discrimination). They would also need to depend on an index of economywide earnings growth. Thus, such a scheme would necessarily be at least as complicated and require at least as much overhead as the current Social Security system, which determines payments based on a beneficiary's age, past earnings, and current labor market earnings, as well as the Consumer Price Index.

The final issue relating to our decomposition of average losses is the choice of comparison group used to estimate lost earnings growth and thus the upper boundaries of regions C, D, and E in figure 7.1. Our preferred loss estimates rely on the average experience of all non-displaced workers to compute lost earnings growth of displaced workers. We also showed in chapters 5 and 6 that basing lost earnings growth estimates only on the experiences of nondisplaced workers from the same firms lowers our estimates by approximately 20 percent.[3] Basing estimates of earnings growth on nondisplaced workers in the same industry implies a somewhat smaller drop in our loss estimates. As we argued in chapter 4, however, nondisplaced workers in firms or industries that experience mass layoffs and plant closing may themselves have experienced some earnings losses as the result of the same events that led to job losses. Thus, we feel that our preferred measure best captures the importance of the events that lead to displacement.

We recognize, however, that a hypothetical program fully compensating workers for lost earnings growth would raise some vexing issues if that lost earnings growth was estimated using the experiences of the general workforce. In particular, if a hypothetical assistance program were to provide full compensation to displaced workers but not to their former colleagues who retained their jobs, then workers in firms or industries adversely affected by structural or policy changes would actually prefer to lose their jobs. Alternatively, the perverse incentives entailed by full compensation could be eliminated by also compensating those who keep jobs in distressed firms or industries. However, such a program would be extremely difficult to administer and would probably enjoy little political support.

As we noted, however, loss estimates are 80 percent as large as our preferred estimates when they are based on the experiences of job keepers in affected firms or industries. Because current programs compensate displaced workers for much less than 80 percent of their losses, compensation can be made substantially more generous without generating the kinds of disincentives mentioned above. Put differently, our results indicate that workers who actually lose their jobs suffer losses several times those of workers who retain their jobs in distressed firms and industries. Given resource levels that are likely to be available for assisting displaced workers, policymakers need not fear overcompensating workers or giving them incentives to become displaced.

In addition to detailing the magnitude and persistence of the average worker's losses, the results in this monograph show how those losses vary across workers. One important finding concerns workers who separate from firms that have had stable employment levels. These workers experience substantial short-term losses. But, in contrast to workers leaving distressed firms, in the long term their earnings return to their expected levels. We believe that this recovery results in large part because some of these workers voluntarily separated from their former firms. For this reason we have chosen to emphasize our results for workers who separate amidst mass layoffs and plant closings. We can be confident that nearly all of these workers are displaced for reasons unrelated to their performance on the job.

Consistent with the literature summarized in chapter 2, we find that earnings losses of displaced workers are similar in percentage terms for men and women. Losses vary somewhat more by industry and age. Young workers and those displaced from the primary metals industries had larger preseparation earnings losses. Postdisplacement losses were larger for older workers and for displaced mining and construction, primary metals, and transportation workers. Depending on the comparison group used, estimated losses for financial and services workers were smaller than those of other displaced workers. We also find that losses are greater for workers displaced in already depressed local labor markets. This latter result suggests that it may be especially useful to concentrate resources in localities where unemployment is high.

We also confirm the common finding that displaced workers who are forced to change major industries experience larger losses. For instance, workers whose previous jobs were in the manufacturing sector but whose new jobs were outside that sector experienced losses equal to nearly 40 percent of their previous earnings. By contrast, those who found reemployment in manufacturing experienced losses of only about 20 percent. This finding suggests that job search assistance programs could have significant value when they help workers find jobs in similar industries. However, our study also shows that even workers who find new jobs in the same narrowly defined (4-digit SIC) industry experience large and persistent losses. Because job search assistance is not likely to do better than to return workers to their old industry, this result suggests that, though it can be valuable, it cannot possibly eliminate their losses.

Overall, we are struck more by the similarities than by the differences in the pattern of losses across groups of workers. Large losses were not limited to older workers or workers from trade-sensitive durable goods industries. Younger workers and workers from the wholesale and retail trade sectors also experienced substantial postdisplacement earnings losses. The pervasiveness of losses implies that the special assistance received by certain classes of workers, such as those deemed to have lost their jobs because of import competition, is not justified by any special difficulties of adjustment. If a concern for fairness motivates policymakers to aid displaced workers, policies should be more broadly targeted and not be restricted to those adversely affected by import competition. Of course, if their motivation for assisting displaced workers is smoothing the way for freer trade, their special concern for trade-impacted workers makes sense.

The pervasiveness of losses also suggests they are not simply the result of the loss of union wage premiums or efficiency wages in particular industries. Instead, because displaced workers from so many demographic groups, industries, and geographic regions experience large earnings losses, our findings suggest that whenever high-tenure workers are displaced, some highly firm-specific attribute of their former employment relationship is lost. The best evidence for this contention is the result mentioned above that even workers who find jobs in the same narrowly defined industry experience substantial earnings losses. If it is workers' skills that are lost, these skills must be firm-specific as opposed to merely industry-specific. Alternatively, earnings losses may result from the workings of internal labor markets. In either case, subsidized training programs cannot directly replace the lost resource and must greatly raise workers' general skills in order to compensate them for their losses.

Finally, our findings also demonstrate the advantages of basing research on long earnings histories for large samples of displaced and nondisplaced workers. From such data, we document: (1) substantial losses even before workers leave their firms, (2) slow earnings recovery, and (3) faster earnings growth among nondisplaced workers in prosperous versus distressed firms. Our results using these administrative data also indicate that previous studies have probably underestimated the earnings losses associated with worker displacement.

7.2 Implications for Traditional Programs

In this section we offer more detailed observations about our study's implications for existing programs that assist displaced workers. As we have noted, such assistance comes in several forms. First, income replacement is available to displaced workers while they are unemployed. This is provided to the general population of job losers by the UI system, while the TAA program provides more extensive benefits to selected displaced workers. Second, workers receive assistance in finding new work. In particular, state ES offices act as a labor exchange for all unemployed workers, while EDWAA provides more extensive services to displaced workers. These services include counseling and formal job search assistance. Third, subsidized training is available to some displaced workers through EDWAA and until recently through the Pell Grant program. Finally, policymakers have endeavored to help displaced workers by mandating advance notice before layoffs and establishing programs to help communities deal with and perhaps forestall large layoffs. We discuss each of these programs below.

The income replacement that the UI system provides to unemployed job losers is the largest component of the safety net that protects workers from the direst consequences of job loss. Each state has considerable discretion in structuring its own UI system, but weekly benefits are usually a little less than 50 percent of a worker's previous weekly earnings up to a maximum benefit that varies among states. Regular UI lasts six months, but its duration may be increased considerably in periods of high unemployment. When the insured unemployment rate (IUR) rises above 6 percent, the Extended Benefit (EB) program provides federal funds to increase the duration of UI payments for an additional 13 weeks. Recently, because of the substantial decline in the ratio between the IUR and the unemployment rate, Congress established a series of temporary Emergency Unemployment Benefit (EUB) programs to provide extended benefits to qualified unemployed workers.

The decline in the ratio of insured to total unemployment reflects an increase in the number of unemployed workers who do not file claims for UI. Indeed, in our sample of high-tenure workers separating from distressed firms, a surprisingly high 40 percent did not receive any UI benefits. The large number of unemployed workers not receiving UI benefits has caused some policymakers to be concerned that eligibility standards have become overly restrictive. However, in our sample only a handful of the 40 percent of workers who did not claim benefits had as much as one quarter without any earnings. This suggests that many displaced workers do not file for benefits simply because they do not have a difficult time finding new jobs. Of course, our results imply that they do have a difficult time finding new jobs that pay as much as their old ones.

Another trend that has concerned policymakers has been the increase in the fraction of workers collecting UI benefits who subsequently exhaust those benefits. Indeed, in our sample of displaced workers this fraction is approximately 56 percent. Thus, many displaced workers appear to have difficult transitions to new employment. This high fraction of workers exhausting benefits has been argued by many to imply a need to extend the normal length of benefits. However, as we have noted, extending the duration of benefits may significantly delay reemployment and thus may be costly to the economy. More effective means of aiding the unemployed or speeding their returns to work would clearly be valuable.

TAA is another form of extended UI that provides workers with up to 52 weeks of additional benefits. To receive TAA, however, a petition must be filed with the Department of Labor demonstrating that job loss resulted from import competition. This requirement greatly limits the number of workers eligible for help. As we noted above, these special benefits are not, in general, justified by any special difficulties trade-impacted workers face because of their job losses. Rather, our results indicate that large losses are the rule for all high-tenure displaced workers. An additional feature of TAA is that receipt of benefits for the maximum duration is tied to the use of a voucher, worth up to $10,000, to pay for training services. As we argue below, this probably does not lead to an efficient use of resources.

An important implication of our results is that because only a small portion of earnings losses accrue while workers are unemployed, the benefits UI and TAA provide are small compared to the magnitude of losses. We can demonstrate this directly by recomputing workers' losses on the basis of their incomes, including their receipt of UI and TAA. Figure 7.2 displays this recomputation of losses for the mass layoff sample of chapter 6. Also shown are the losses we previously computed strictly on the basis of wage and salary earnings. As can be seen in the figure, UI and TAA reduce earnings losses by only a relatively small amount and only in the quarters surrounding job separations. This finding reflects the requirement that workers must be unemployed to receive UI and TAA, that these programs replace less than 50 percent of predisplacement wages, and that payments usually last less than six months. Clearly, income replacement programs ease the transition to lower earnings by reducing the large losses in the year after separation, but in the long run they have no impact on living standards of displaced workers.[4]

Despite the fact that they compensate for only a small portion of losses, UI and TAA may significantly decrease incentives to return to work. Although the UI system usually replaces no more than 50 percent of previous earnings, our results indicate that it often replaces a much larger fraction of earnings on subsequent jobs. For example, in states with high UI benefits, displaced workers who previously earned $16 per hour, would qualify for benefits paying the equivalent of $7.50 per hour for a 40-hour week. Our results suggest that the average displaced worker would be hard pressed to find a new job with starting pay much above $10 per hour. Because the UI and TAA benefits represent such a large fraction of what they could earn by working, some displaced workers will prefer to remain unemployed and receive benefits rather than return to work. In addition, EB, EUB, and TAA programs that extend the duration of benefits are likely to further increase durations of unemployment.

Figure 7.2   Losses of Earnings and Losses of Income (Earnings Plus UI and TAA Payments) of Mass Layoff Separators

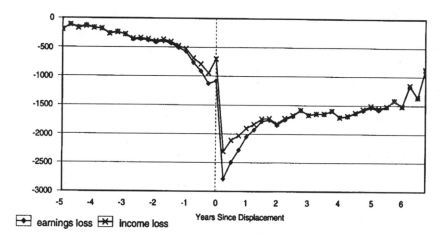

These results may shed some light on the findings of other studies that one of the most important reasons for the significant rise in unemployment rates since the 1960s has been a rise in unemployment durations, particularly for prime-age men (Murphy and Topel 1987). High-tenure, prime-age workers appear to be more likely to lose their jobs than in the past, and such workers have longer durations of unemployment than other workers. Moreover, the interaction between the size of these workers' earnings losses and the parameters of the UI system likely further increases the length of their average unemployment spells.

Because programs that offer weekly cash payments to unemployed workers retard adjustment, several states have experimented with offering reemployment bonuses to encourage UI recipients' rapid return to work. In these state demonstrations, workers received lump-sum payments if they found jobs within a specified period following job loss. In effect, these payments allowed unemployed workers to receive some compensation even after they returned to work. Evaluations of these experimental programs indicate that bonuses modestly reduce time unemployed without increasing the costs of state UI programs or lowering subsequent wages.[5] In the context of the present UI system, however, it is clear that the more rapid reemployment they encourage would have scant impact on the losses incurred by displaced workers. However, if displaced workers were to be offered UI benefits of substantially greater potential duration, the value of reemployment bonus programs might be greatly increased.

Policymakers also have taken steps to help displaced workers find new employment. First, each state administers a federally funded Employment Service that acts as a labor exchange matching unemployed workers to employer job vacancies. As a condition for receiving their benefits, UI recipients are required to register with their state ES. Thus the ES comes into contact with a great many workers making difficult transitions to new employment. The effectiveness of the ES has been questioned, however, because states place only about 6 percent of their registrants, and most of those workers are placed in low-wage jobs. Nevertheless, two studies (Johnson et al. 1986; and Katz 1990) suggest that although its cost is low, the ES is a useful resource for those who fail to find jobs through friends and relatives, direct applications at work sites, or other channels. As a result, the ES cost effectively reduces the time these registrants spend unemployed.

The modest achievements of the ES may simply reflect the modest resources devoted to it. Unfortunately, federal funds for the ES system are currently less than 75 percent of the per registrant levels of 1980. This has caused state ESs to largely terminate counseling and testing services that were once widely available. As a result many states have begun to use their own funds to enhance job search assistance. Further, as we discuss below, several states have combined ES funds with those provided by other federal programs and used their ES as the lead agency in a combined program. Greater funding for this modest but cost-effective program seems to us to be a good investment.

In addition to the services of the ES, which are available to all unemployed workers, policymakers have provided special readjustment assistance to displaced workers. The primary federal legislation authorizing the provision of such services is the Economic Dislocation and Worker Adjustment Assistance Act. This legislation amended Title III of the Job Training Partnership Act (JTPA). Under this act, the JTPA programs targeted toward the economically disadvantaged as well as the services targeted toward displaced workers are run locally by Private Industry Councils. Despite its name, eligibility for EDWAA services is not limited to recently displaced workers, but also extends to the long-term unemployed. Thus eligibility for EDWAA services theoretically extends to perhaps millions of workers per year. In reality, however, funding constraints have limited participation to about 120,000 workers annually.[6]

EDWAA provides its clients with a diverse set of services. On average, their participation lasts 14 weeks. During this time, displaced workers receive job search assistance and possibly on-the-job or classroom training. In addition, EDWAA provides for a rapid response service, usually run at the state level. This service is designed to counsel recently laid-off workers about alternative programs and to help them develop realistic adjustment plans. Policymakers intend that these services will prevent participants from becoming discouraged or from developing overly optimistic expectations about wages at available jobs.

Previous research has found job search assistance of the kind provided by EDWAA to be highly cost effective. In the past, these relatively inexpensive programs have quickened displaced workers' return to work and raised at least their short-term earnings. Though it is highly cost effective, it should be emphasized that previous research also shows that job search assistance can only alleviate a small portion of earnings losses of the magnitude that we document.

The limited effectiveness of job search assistance programs should not be surprising, because the results in this monograph indicate that a significant portion of the earnings losses of displaced workers result from the loss of some firm-specific attribute of the former employment relationship. No matter how good job search programs are at placing displaced workers in new jobs, our results indicate that long-term earnings losses will still average 15 to 20 percent. However, our findings suggest that the cost effectiveness of job search assistance might be enhanced if it concentrated on placing manufacturing workers who would have wound up in the nonmanufacturing sector back into the manufacturing sector. Counseling and relocation assistance also might enhance the effectiveness of these programs.

The inability of public sector-supported job search to substantially reduce displaced worker earnings has induced policymakers to increase their emphasis on retraining programs. Such programs are designed to raise the long-term earnings of displaced workers by enhancing their marketable skills. In fact, approximately one-third of EDWAA enrollees receive such classroom instruction, usually lasting approximately 30 weeks. This retraining is provided in special classes run almost exclusively by local community colleges and vocational-technical schools. Classes are more intensive than ordinary community college classes, and students usually receive significantly more support services. These services include matching courses both to local job opportunities and to the workers' aptitudes and interests, as well as enhanced placement services.

Unfortunately, the program evaluation literature provides little reason for optimism about the ability of federally sponsored training programs to substantially reduce long-term losses. For instance, in a survey of training programs for the displaced, Leigh (1990) concluded that "there is no clear evidence that either classroom training or on-the-job training has a significant impact on employment or earnings." Indeed, the existing evidence suggests that it is rare for a training program to raise even short-term earnings by $1,000 per year. Such a gain would amount to about one-sixth of displaced workers' annual long-term losses. Moreover, the scant evidence on long-term gains from training programs gives little hope that these short-term gains rise significantly over time.

In determining the mix of services to provide under a program such as EDWAA with its nearly unlimited numbers of potential clients but very limited funding, policymakers face an inevitable choice between breadth and depth. In practice, this amounts to choosing between providing relatively basic and inexpensive job search assistance to large numbers of workers or providing much more expensive job training to a smaller number of workers. This choice ought to depend on the relative rates of return job search assistance and training provide in the form of increased earnings on subsequent jobs, as well as on what would contribute to greater equity among workers.

Our reading of the available evidence strongly suggests that job search assistance has a much higher rate of return than training. In fact, earnings gains from job search assistance are usually as large as those received from training, but the cost of job search assistance is only a fraction of that of training. Moreover, concentration on job search assistance would allow more workers to be served and hence seems more equitable as well. Thus, we regard as unfortunate the stipulation in EDWAA's enabling legislation that half of all funds be spent on classroom training.

The recent New Jersey Unemployment Insurance Reemployment Demonstration (Corson et al. 1989) is especially informative about the relative merits of training and job search assistance. This demonstration used an experimental design to study the incentives of the unemployment insurance system and whether mandatory job search assistance and referrals to JTPA for retraining reduced unemployment durations and raised participants' earnings. The demonstration targeted UI claimants more than 25 years old, who had at least three years' tenure with their former employer and who had been laid off without a recall date for more than four weeks. The demonstration required a random sample of this group to participate in a two-week job search assistance workshop. Afterwards, random sample of these participants was referred to JTPA.

The evaluation indicated that job search assistance raised participants' earnings by $450 during the year after participating in the workshops. However, the opportunity to participate in training apparently did not improve participants' labor market prospects. The earnings gains for those who received both job search assistance and retraining referrals were actually smaller than for those who received only job search assistance. To make the case for retraining even worse, job search assistance cost only a few hundred dollars per participant, whereas the classroom instruction cost $3,100 (1990 dollars) per participant and the on-the-job training cost $2,300 per participant.

The evidence indicates that existing training programs do not significantly reduce the earnings losses of displaced workers. Nevertheless, it is instructive to ask how much might it cost for a hypothetical retraining program to eliminate their $6,000 annual long-term earnings losses. Suppose that a training program is able to generate a 12 percent rate of return on its investment. That return would be high compared to investments in other forms of human capital, such as schooling. However, such a retraining program could generate a permanent earnings gain of $6,000 per year only at a cost of $50,000. This figure would correspond to a program that required participants to spend two years out of the labor force, thereby foregoing $15,000 - $19,000 per year in lost earnings in a full-time retraining program with direct costs of $6,000 - $10,000 per year. Such a program would be equivalent to paying the tuition, books, and other expenses so that a displaced worker could go back to school full time to acquire an Associates degree. Notice that this program, like the existing EDWAA program, does not include any stipend to cover living expenses.

Until recently, the Pell Grant program also provided assistance to large numbers of displaced workers seeking retraining. A special provision of that program waived the normal limit on students' prior year income for displaced workers, allowing them to receive grants for full-time postsecondary education.[7] During the 1990-91 academic year, over 75,000 displaced workers received Pell Grants, 5 percent more than attended classroom training under EDWAA. We know of no research formally evaluating the ability of the Pell Grant program to raise the earnings of displaced workers, but its approach seems to us to have had some advantages over the provision of training under EDWAA. One advantage of the Pell Grant approach is that workers had a wider choice of educational programs. For example, approximately 30 percent of displaced workers receiving Pell Grants attended proprietary schools and another 10 percent attended four-year colleges where instruction is usually more intensive than at the community colleges where EDWAA training is provided. It is also likely that Pell grantees, who usually paid a substantial portion of schooling costs themselves, were more motivated learners than workers whose attendance at training programs is required as a condition for continued receipt of TAA payments. Thus, it was probably unfortunate that the special provision for displaced workers was eliminated when the Higher Education Act was reauthorized in 1992.

Another source of support for displaced workers is the federally mandated requirement that firms with 100 or more employees give workers 60 days advance notice of a plant closing or any layoff involving more than one-third of their workforce. This mandate is intended to give workers time to develop adjustment strategies and, perhaps more important, to give local governments time to ready appropriate services. Our results demonstrate that high-tenure workers covered by the law are still likely to experience long-term earnings losses resulting from their job losses.

While a consensus on the effectiveness of this mandate has yet to develop, some studies suggest that early notification helps reduce the time spent unemployed following job loss (Ruhm 1992). However, given the large and long-lasting losses of these workers after they find new jobs, it is hard to imagine how 60 days or even six months advance notice would have any appreciable impact on reducing earnings losses. Moreover, because such a large fraction of earnings loss is related to the loss of some attribute of the employment relationship, even if, as some studies argue, advance notice eases the transition to new jobs requiring similar skills, substantial losses would remain. In addition, our findings showing substantial preseparation earnings losses indicate that even without formal notice, workers have information indicating that hard times lie ahead. These considerations indicate that, although early notification laws single out workers likely to experience substantial losses, the notification itself is probably of little practical value in reducing the long-term earnings losses of high-tenure workers.

There are at least three further steps that can be taken at the federal level to improve the functioning of programs to aid displaced workers. The first step is to concentrate resources so states can effectively coordinate programs. Currently, there are 125 separate programs providing retraining to various groups of workers.[8] Coordinating these programs at the state level is very difficult because each program imposes different requirements for receiving aid, enrolling participants, tracking progress, and reporting results. Because the thrusts of the programs are similar, it often would require relatively little change to institute a common set of requirements and avoid needless duplication.

A second step that could be taken at the federal level would be to foster federal-state cooperation in tracking program participation and performance. This cooperation probably could best be achieved by establishing a common set of criteria for collecting relevant data. Such a system would provide information on participants, services provided, and outcomes 13 weeks following job loss. Longer term follow-up also would be possible by linking participant records with the same state UI earnings and firm records used for this analysis. Such a data collection system for displaced workers could be modeled on the U.S. Department of Labor's new data collection system for tracking economically disadvantaged workers in JTPA Title IIA programs. This system has established a common set of tracking forms across the more than 600 Service Delivery Areas and has the resulting data electronically transmitted to a central depository in each state and then to a federal data center.

Finally, federal and state governments should continue to explore the feasibility and effectiveness of programs that help firms and employees develop plans that either forestall mass layoffs or ease the transition of displaced workers to new employment. In Canada, the Industrial Assistance Service performs this function by helping interested parties establish management-labor committees and providing them with technical assistance and "honest brokers." One component of these services assists the committees in addressing problems associated with plant closings. In the U.S., this component of the Canadian program has recently been tested in a demonstration run jointly by the Department of Labor and the National Governors Association.

A related model for dealing with plant closings comes from the Community Adjustment Program established by the U.S. Department of Defense. Because military facilities closures impose large costs on affected communities, this program turns closed facilities over to the community for a minimal charge and develops an economic plan for the facility's civilian use. Examples of such conversions are the commercial airport in Bangor, Maine and the Fort Custer Industrial Park in Battle Creek, Michigan. Although little is known about the benefits of these industrial assistance programs, two advantages in their favor are that they are relatively inexpensive and that they do not provide substantial government subsidies to inefficient firms.

In conclusion, the existing array of programs designed to aid displaced workers provides modest short-term relief but does little to reduce long-term losses. No existing program provides the costly, long-lasting assistance that could conceivably come close to fully offsetting these losses. Moreover, though we believe that current programs could be improved through reorganization and in some cases additional funding, it is doubtful whether they ever could fully restore the lost earnings potential of displaced workers.

7.3 Implications for a Wage Subsidy Program

In this section we offer some more speculative thoughts on alternative programs that would provide greater levels of compensation to displaced workers by continuing to supplement their incomes beyond the period of their unemployment. In contrast to traditional employment and training programs, the programs we discuss in this section would make no pretense of increasing worker productivity. Instead, they would simply transfer income from the beneficiaries of technological or policy changes to those harmed by these events. We have already discussed the varied rationales for such a policy and observed that existing programs under UI and EDWAA only compensate the displaced for a small fraction of their losses. Our purpose here is to discuss the implications of our findings for the design of programs that would more fully compensate displaced workers.

Recall that this study contains several findings that are particularly relevant to the design of programs intended to reduce earnings losses. First, because quarterly losses persist, workers' cumulative losses are extremely large. Second, the bulk of these losses accrue after workers are reemployed and not during prolonged or frequent periods of unemployment following their displacements. Third, because the UI system replaces roughly 40 to 50 percent of predisplacement earnings and because displacement substantially lowers earnings prospects, UI benefits are likely to be a relatively large percentage of earnings from postdisplacement jobs. Finally, workers who remained employed in distressed firms also experience modest losses.

The severity of displaced worker losses implies that the annual costs of a program that fully compensated them would be substantial even if participation in such a program were limited to experienced workers like those studied in this monograph. Our estimate that 2.6 million such workers were displaced nationwide during the seven-year period studied suggests an annual average of 350,000 such displacements. At a loss of $80,000 per worker, the cost of making them "whole" would amount to approximately $26 billion annually. Alternatively, if policymakers were to bring the incomes of displaced workers only up to the level of the nondisplaced workers in their former firms, the estimated budget cost falls by 20 percent to $20 billion. Even this latter figure is several times larger than current expenditures on displaced workers. Thus, given the current political climate, it seems very unlikely that policymakers would implement a program that came close to making displaced workers whole.

Still, the gap between earnings losses and current levels of assistance is so large that policymakers may be inclined to design alternative programs that provide substantially more generous assistance to the displaced. If such programs are to avoid unnecessary inefficiencies, they will need to pay attention to two sometimes conflicting goals: First, they will want to target the assistance they provide toward those who have suffered the greatest losses. Second, they will want to insure that workers have incentives to find new and better-paying jobs.

The conflict that sometimes emerges between these two goals can be seen in the alternative designs proposed for the basic UI system. The current system pays weekly benefits as long as workers remain unemployed up to some maximum duration. This design makes sense from the point of view of targeting the most assistance toward workers who have the most difficult transitions, since workers who are unemployed longer tend to both have more difficult transitions and to receive the most assistance from UI. However, the current system reduces the incentives of the unemployed to find jobs because they stop receiving benefits once they are reemployed. As we have noted, the UI system creates especially strong disincentives for displaced workers of the kind studied to return to work. On average, regular UI benefits might be as much as 75 percent of what such workers could expect to earn on their next job, and for some workers, UI benefits may exceed the wages they could earn in the labor market.

Because regular weekly UI benefits embody incentives that delay the return to work, an alternative design has been proposed in which a single "lump-sum" payment is given to workers when they lose their jobs. Such a payment could directly compensate displaced workers for a portion of their expected losses, much the way a "back pay" award compensates a plaintiff in a wrongful discharge case. The primary advantage of providing permanently dislocated workers with a single lump-sum payment is that this compensation does not depend on whether they find work. As a result they have no incentive to remain unemployed. An additional advantage of this design is that it does not require administrators to follow displaced workers over an extended period of time.

A program in which all displaced workers received a single lump-sum payment does not, however, satisfy the objective of targeting the most assistance toward those who have the most need. The problem is that such a program not only compensates dislocated workers who have difficulty adjusting to their job losses, but also those who adjust relatively easily to their displacements. For example, under this scheme a worker who found a new job immediately after his layoff would receive just as much compensation as a worker who took an entire year to find new employment. If a significant percentage of all displaced workers do not experience difficult transitions, the cost of a program based on single lump-sum payments would be greater than necessary to achieve the objective of providing reasonable compensation for earnings losses.

The reemployment bonus experiments discussed in the previous section can be viewed as a compromise between a lump-sum scheme and a traditional UI system that attempts to meet both objectives—targeting resources on those most in need and providing incentives to return to work—reasonably well. Recall that in these designs, when unemployed workers find new jobs by a certain date, they are entitled to a cash payment. This cash payment or bonus provides workers with a clear incentive to return to work by the specified date. As an addition to the present UI system, these bonuses have been shown to modestly reduce unemployment spell lengths without reducing wages on subsequent jobs.

The increased incentives that bonus programs provide for the unemployed to return to work might be an especially useful component of a program that attempted to more generously assist displaced workers by extending the duration of their UI benefits, as is presently done with TAA. Without reemployment bonuses, such an extension would increase compensation to the displaced, but at the cost of worsening their reemployment incentives. Incorporating bonuses into a program with longer maximum benefit durations might have a bigger impact on incentives for the displaced to find new work. Indeed, some evidence exists from the Illinois reemployment bonus experiment that these payments were more effective when claimants were eligible for 38 rather than 26 weeks of benefits (Decker, O'Leary, and Woodbury 1993).

While bonus programs provide workers with better incentives to return to work than the standard UI system, they also target assistance toward those most in need better than a pure lump-sum system. The bonus is, of course, a kind of lump-sum payment received even by workers who have little difficulty finding new jobs. However, it is smaller than the lump sums that would be paid under a pure lump-sum scheme. Moreover, while under a pure lump-sum scheme all displaced workers receive compensation, under a bonus scheme workers must file a claim for UI and, depending on the program, perhaps remain unemployed a few weeks, before receiving a bonus. This extra hurdle imposed by the bonus scheme keeps some workers who do not face difficult transitions from collecting benefits. Of course, its importance would depend on the size of the bonus, with higher bonuses inducing more workers who don't expect difficulty in finding new work to participate in the program. However, as long as bonuses remain smaller than pure lump-sum payments, bonus schemes will have more success targeting workers most in need of help.

The reason the lump-sum and the UI reemployment bonus schemes increase incentives to return to work is that these programs allow workers to receive compensation without remaining unemployed. This also could be accomplished by offering workers cash payments or tax credits in the form of income or earnings subsidies after they return to work (Lerman 1982). Tying the level of assistance to incomes or earnings levels on subsequent jobs would also allow policymakers to better target assistance toward those who suffer the greatest losses. If earnings always returned to their predisplacement levels, then the number of weeks workers spent unemployed would be a reliable indicator of the severity of their losses. But, our results show that the biggest portion of their losses actually occur in the form of lower earnings after they return to work. Thus, the number of weeks workers spend unemployed may be only loosely related to the ultimate size of their losses. In contrast, an earnings subsidy that is larger for workers with larger earnings declines would allow assistance to be matched much more closely to losses. This suggests that an earnings subsidy program may work well by the criteria of both incentives and targeting.

The most ambitious form of an income or earnings subsidy program would be one designed to make workers whole by paying them the difference between their actual earnings and their expected earnings had the events that caused their displacements not occurred. In order to make workers truly whole, these payments would have to begin while workers were unemployed and their actual earnings were zero. Moreover, workers would need to receive a one-time payment for the portion of their losses that occurred before actual separation. Unfortunately, as we observed earlier, such a program would be prohibitively costly. Another problem with this design is that it would be difficult to administer because, as this study demonstrated, it is difficult to compute "expected" earnings. In particular, such a computation would require subsidy payments to depend on workers' age, sex, and earnings histories, as well as an aggregate index of economywide earnings growth.

More important, this highly ambitious earnings subsidy program would fail at providing workers with incentives to find new and higher-paying jobs. Under this hypothetical program, workers whose earnings would have been expected to grow would receive more than 100 percent of their previous earnings while unemployed. Because we found that, on average, their earnings on subsequent jobs were 25 percent lower, this would correspond to approximately 125 percent of what they could expect to earn by taking a job. Moreover, even if they were to take a new job, the program would not provide them with the proper incentives to work more hours or find better jobs. As long as they remained below the earnings levels expected prior to their displacements, they would receive no benefit from higher earnings. Rather, each dollar of higher earnings would be offset by a dollar less of earnings subsidy. The severe work disincentives generated by such a program would undoubtedly greatly lower displaced workers' earnings and increase costs even more than the estimates presented above.

Though an earnings subsidy that makes workers whole would clearly be bad policy, a modified version might be worth consideration. First, in order to make the program less administratively burdensome, subsidy levels could be based on predisplacement earnings levels rather than postdisplacement levels expected before displacement occurred. Earnings up to three years prior to separation could be used to calculate a reasonable predisplacement earnings level which could then be indexed to the Consumer Price Index to prevent inflation from shrinking the size of the benefit. Second, in order to give workers the incentive to return to work, the subsidy could be restricted to employed workers. Finally, in order to give workers the incentive to earn more by working longer hours and finding better jobs, the subsidy could be reduced in such a way as to eliminate the implicit 100 percent tax rate. For example, the wage subsidy program could (1) pay a subsidy equal to 40 percent of earnings to a worker who earned 30 percent or less of predislocation wages, and (2) reduce this subsidy by four-sevenths of a dollar for each dollar of earnings above 30 percent. According to this design, the subsidy would decline from 40 percent to 0 percent of predisplacement earnings as postdisplacement wages rose from 30 percent to 100 percent of their predisplacement levels. Each of these changes also would reduce the subsidy's cost.

Table 7.1 shows the subsidy levels that a worker whose predisplacement earnings were $24,000 would receive under such a program for various postdisplacement earnings levels. For example, if earnings on a new job were $7,200, or 30 percent of predisplacement earnings, the third column of the table shows that the worker would receive an earnings subsidy of $9,600, or 40 percent of predisplacement earnings. As the fourth column shows, this would bring total income to $16,800. The last column of the table shows that the worker's income would still be $7,200 per year less than predisplacement earnings. If the postdisplacement earnings were less than 30 percent of predisplacement earnings, the worker would still receive the same $9,600 subsidy, but if earnings exceeded $7,200, the subsidy would be decreased. For example, if postdisplacement earnings were to increase to $12,000, or 50 percent of predisplacement earnings, the subsidy would decline to $6,857. But, in contrast to the case of the hypothetical subsidy that makes workers whole, his or her total income would increase to $18,857. This pattern of decreasing subsidies and increasing total income would continue until the worker's earnings matched the predisplacement level of $24,000. At that point the worker would stop receiving subsidies.

Table 7.1 Income Support in a Hypothetical Earnings Subsidy Scheme When Predisplacement Earnings Were $24,000

Postdisplacement earnings	Percentage of predisplacement earnings	Annual subsidy	Total annual income	Uncompensated annual earnings decline
$4,800	20	$9,600	$14,400	$9,600
7,200	30	9,600	16,800	7,200
9,600	40	8,229	17,829	6,171
12,000	50	6,857	18,857	5,143
14,400	60	5,486	19,886	4,114
16,800	70	4,114	20,914	3,086
19,200	80	2,743	21,943	2,057
21,600	90	1,371	22,971	1,029
24,000	100	0	24,000	—
26,400	110	0	26,400	—

The modified version of the earnings subsidy described above provides substantial incentives for displaced workers to find new jobs and once reemployed to continue to increase their earnings. For example, if the hypothetical worker whose predisplacement earnings were $24,000 was receiving UI benefits, he or she would have an income on an annual basis of approximately $12,000. Table 7.1 shows that even if the worker took a job paying half of his or her old earnings level, the total annual income would be almost $19,000. Moreover, if, as would be reasonably likely, the worker found a job paying 80 percent of the old level, total annual income would be nearly $22,500, or $10,500 above what would be obtained by collecting UI. These income increases over the levels provided by UI should induce displaced workers to find new work. Under the modified earnings subsidy, each $1,000 increase in earnings would increase income by at least $430, so workers would also have reasonable incentives to work harder and earn more.

Though it provides strong work incentives, the modified earnings subsidy program would still target those in need better than the current UI system. On the one hand, workers able to quickly find new jobs paying wages comparable to those of their old jobs would have no strong incentive to claim UI benefits and would receive little or no assistance from the earnings subsidy program. On the other hand, workers who quickly find new jobs but experience large earnings declines would receive a greater share of the available resources than under the current UI system. Since our results suggest that such workers experience a large share of the cumulative losses, this program would improve targeting.

To arrive at some crude estimates of the likely costs of such an earnings subsidy, consider the figures in table 7.1. A worker whose postdisplacement earnings were $19,200 or 80 percent of predisplacement earnings would receive a subsidy of approximately $2,700 per year. By contrast, a worker displaced into a job paying near the minimum wage would receive a subsidy exceeding $9,000 annually. Because the former case is more typical of the experiences of high-tenure workers, it is reasonable to use the $2,700 figure as the basis for estimating the likely costs of the wage subsidy program. If these subsidies were paid to displaced workers for the rest of their working lives, such a program would cost approximately $9 billion annually.

(This amount assumes that each year under the existing UI system there will be 350,000 new displaced eligible persons who receive an average of $2,700 over the rest of their working lives.) Of course, these costs could be lowered if policymakers chose to limit the number of years that displaced workers were eligible to receive the subsidy. For example, if the subsidy lasted only two years beyond the date of displaced workers' UI claims, the annual costs would fall to less than $2 billion.

The foregoing cost estimates of a wage subsidy are meant to be illustrative. Actual program estimates will depend on more factors than addressed here. For example, depending on how they are designed, earnings subsidies will affect the costs of the UI system by altering participation rates and the duration of benefits. In addition, other cost considerations include the movement of real wages and the age of displaced workers. When real wages are growing, a wage subsidy like that described above is less costly because postdisplacement wages are more likely to exceed predisplacement wages. Likewise, younger workers are less costly to serve than their older counterparts because their wage growth is usually faster. Unfortunately, real wages have been declining for two decades and the workforce is aging. These trends serve to raise the cost of a wage subsidy. Nevertheless, the crude estimates presented in this section suggest that there are feasible alternatives to existing policies that would provide increased support for those most adversely affected by displacement, while preserving strong work incentives.

To be sure, our cost estimates for an earnings subsidy program are substantial compared to current outlays, even when the subsidy only lasts two years. However, compared to the likely gains received by the rest of society from many technology or policy changes, these costs are small. For example, some studies indicate that ratification of the North American Free Trade Agreement (NAFTA) would raise U.S. GDP by approximately 1 percent or $60 billion per year. In this light, a program that annually transfers $2 to $3 billion to displaced workers in industries adversely affected by NAFTA would appear to be a reasonable concession to those fearing the treaty's adverse consequences. Indeed, if NAFTA's advocates believe that the treaty will greatly benefit the U.S. economy, they should endorse such a subsidy simply because it would substantially raise the likelihood of the treaty's passage.

7.4 Summary

Our finding that displaced workers from a wide array of industries and demographic groups incur large and persistent losses demonstrates the substantial value of the employment relationship to experienced workers. For such workers, job loss is equivalent in financial terms to losing an $80,000 home in a natural disaster such as a hurricane or flood. Put this way, it is easy to understand why policymakers often fail to enact policies such as trade liberalization that bring society net benefits even though they threaten worker displacement. The problem is that while the benefits of such policies are divided among the many who enjoy lower prices for the goods they buy, the costs are borne mainly by the relatively few who lose their jobs. This unequal division of the costs and benefits of productive change strikes many as unfair. Even those immune to appeals to fairness should, however, be concerned about the plight of the displaced, because in our political system a minority for whom an issue is particularly salient can often prevail over a majority for whom an issue is a lesser priority. Trade liberalization and similar policies may be good for society as a whole, but enacting them is likely to be politically impossible if too many workers fear displacement.

Our results also show that the existing programs designed to assist job losers do little to reduce fear of displacement because they do little to reduce the associated losses. Unemployment insurance, the major form of assistance received by displaced workers, only replaces a portion of their earnings and only for the relatively short period they are unemployed. It does nothing to eliminate the majority of their loss, which our results show accumulates in the form of lower earnings on subsequent jobs. Other programs also have limited abilities to help displaced workers. For instance, while low-cost job search assistance programs have been shown to be highly cost effective, the best they probably can do is help workers find similar jobs. Our results, however, show that even workers finding jobs in the same narrowly defined industry experience large losses, implying definite limits to the potential effectiveness of job search. The prospects for eliminating losses through worker retraining programs are even bleaker, since research has shown that training displaced workers often generates low returns. Moreover, even if the returns to retraining were comparable to those of other investments in human capital, significantly reducing a displaced worker's losses would require about the equivalent of two years of college education. So far, however, policymakers have been willing to provide only about the equivalent of a few months of summer school.

We have noted a number of steps that could be taken to increase the effectiveness of current assistance efforts. For instance, though UI does relatively little to lessen displacement's impact, it probably serves to delay reemployment, since many workers must ultimately accept jobs that pay little more than their weekly benefit levels. A program of reemployment bonuses is likely to be especially effective for such workers. A thorough reorganization that eliminated duplication and instituted common eligibility requirements for the more than 125 separate assistance efforts would lower costs as well as make getting help less frustrating for displaced workers. Such a reorganization should probably include a coordinating role and more funding for state ES offices. The effectiveness of these agencies has been challenged without compelling evidence. Most important, the resources EDWAA currently devotes to providing classroom training to a relatively small number of workers could almost certainly be better employed providing low-cost job search assistance to all who could benefit. This would generate greater aggregate earnings improvements as well as increase equity. If these steps were taken, the burden placed on displaced workers could be lessened with relatively little cost. Even with these steps, however, it is clear that displacement will continue to be a major financial setback for workers, one whose prospect will fiercely be resisted.

If policymakers were to act to provide displaced workers with substantially more generous assistance, we have argued that an earnings or income subsidy may be a good way to deliver it. Under such a plan, earnings on new jobs would be supplemented with payments that would depend on how much earnings had declined from previous levels. Such a program could provide generous help to those suffering large losses without at the same time transferring large sums to workers who do not experience major losses. Moreover, such a subsidy could be designed to give the displaced strong incentives to return to work and, once reemployed, to continue to increase their earnings. Ultimately, the decision to adopt an earnings subsidy or some other more generous assistance program will depend on the largely normative and political rationales discussed above. Providing greater compensation to displaced workers may be attractive on grounds of fairness and equity. It may also be a prerequisite to productive change.

NOTES

1. This is most common in macroeconomic discussions of the "trade-off" between inflation and unemployment. If the unemployment in question consists entirely of temporary layoffs, this focus on the unemployment rate may be appropriate. But if the unemployment which is traded for lower inflation consists in part of permanent job losses, then our results imply that the unemployment rate is far from an adequate summary of the costs of more stable prices.

2. Including the preseparation losses in the total of losses due to unemployment does not significantly change our conclusion that losses due to unemployment are a small fraction of total losses.

3. This estimate can only be made for workers whose former firms remained in existence.

4. Sources of income not included in figure 7.2 are supplemental unemployment benefits (SUB) and early retirement pensions. SUB were prevalent in the steel industry and may have substantially reduced short-term losses. Pensions had little effect on our analysis because we examined prime-age workers, who usually were not eligible for such benefits.

5. See Woodbury and Spiegelman (1987); Corson et al. (1989); and Davidson and Woodbury (1993).

6. A recent Congressional Budget Office study (1993) notes that funding levels have recently risen to levels consistent with participation of around 200,000 workers per year.

7. Pell Grants are generally available to full-time postsecondary students whose prior year income was below a certain limit. For displaced workers the limit was until recently based on current year income.

8. "Labor Issues," United States General Accounting Office, Office of the Comptroller General, Report No. GAO/OCG-93-19TR, December 1992.

References

Addison, John, and Pedro Portugal. 1989. "Job Displacement, Relative Wage Changes, and Duration of Unemployment," *Journal of Labor Economics* 7, 3: 281-302.

Akerlof, George. 1982. "Labor Contracts as Partial Gift Exchange," *Quarterly Journal of Economics* 100, 3:543-569.

Akerlof, George, and Janet Yellen. 1985. "Unemployment Through the Filter of Memory," *Quarterly Journal of Economics* 100, 3: 747-53.

Anderson, Patricia, and Bruce D. Meyer. 1992. Unpublished mimeo, Northwestern University.

Ashenfelter, Orley. 1978. "Estimating the Effect of Training Programs on Earnings," *Review of Economics and Statistics* 60 (February): 47-57.

Ashenfelter, Orley, and David Card. 1985, "Using the Longitudinal Structure of Earnings to Estimate the Effect of Training Programs," *Review of Economics and Statistics* 67, 4 (November): 648-660.

Bassi, Laurie. 1984. "Estimating the Effects of Training Programs with Nonrandom Selection," *Review of Economics and Statistics* 66 (February): 36-43.

Beaudry, Paul, and John DiNardo. 1989. "Long-Term Contracts and Equilibrium Models of the Labor Market: Some Favorable Evidence." Working Paper No. 252, Industrial Relations Section, Princeton University, May.

————. 1991. "The Effects of Implicit Contracts on the Movements of Wages Over the Business Cycle: Evidence From Micro Data," *Journal of Political Economy* 99, 4: 665-688.

Becker, Gary. 1975. *Human Capital*, 2nd ed. New York: National Bureau of Economic Research.

Blanchflower, David. 1991. "Fear, Unemployment, and Pay Flexibility," *Economic Journal* 101 (May): 483-96.

Blank, Rebecca, and David Card. 1990. "Recent Trends in Insured and Uninsured Unemployment: Is There an Explanation?" *Quarterly Journal of Economics* 106, 4 (November): 1157-89.

Blau, Francine D., and Marianne A. Ferber. 1987. "Discrimination: Empirical Evidence From the United States," *American Economic Review, Papers and Proceedings* 77, 2 (May): 316-320.

Blau, Francine D., and Lawrence Kahn. 1981. "Causes and Consequences of Layoffs," *Economic Inquiry* 19 (April): 209-96.

Bound, John, and Alan Krueger. 1991. "The Extent of Measurement Error in Longitudinal Earnings Data: Do Two Wrongs Make a Right?" *Journal of Labor Economics* 9, 1: 1-24.

174

Card, David, and Daniel Sullivan. 1988. "Measuring the Effects of CETA Participation on Movements In and Out of Employment," *Econometrica* 56, 3: 497-530.

Congressional Budget Office. 1993. "Displaced Workers: Trends in the 1980s and Implications for the Future," February.

Cordes, Joseph, and Burton Weisbrod. 1979. "Governmental Behavior in Response to Compensation Requirements," *Journal of Public Economics* 11: 47-58

Corson, Walter, Shari Dunstan, Paul Decker, and Anne Gordon. 1989. "New Jersey Unemployment Insurance Reemployment Demonstration Project." Unemployment Insurance Occasional Paper 89-3, U.S. Department of Labor.

Corson, Walter, and Walter Nicholson. 1981. "Trade Adjustment Assistance for Workers: Results of a Survey of Recipients Under the Trade Act of 1974." In *Research in Labor Economics*, Vol. 4, Ronald Ehrenberg, ed. Greenwich, CT: JAI Press, pp. 417-469.

Davidson, Carl, and Stephen A. Woodbury. 1992. "The Displacement Effect of Reemployment Bonus Programs." Mimeo, Michigan State University.

Decker, Paul, Christopher O'Leary, and Stephen Woodbury. Forthcoming. "Impacts on Receipt of Unemployment." In *Incentives for Reemployment: Results of Three Field Experiments in Unemployment Insurance,* Robert Spiegelman and Orley Ashenfelter, eds. Kalamazoo, MI: W. E. Upjohn Institute.

Di la Rica, Sara. 1992. "Displaced Workers in Mass Layoffs: Pre-Displacement Earnings Losses and Unions Effect." Working Paper No. 303, Industrial Relations Section, Princeton University.

Economic Commentary. 1992. Federal Bank of Cleveland, October 15.

Economic Report of the President. 1991. Washington, DC: Government Printing Office.

Flaim, Paul, and Ellen Seghal. 1985 "Displaced Workers of 1979 -83: How Well Have They Fared?" Bulletin 2240, U.S. Department of Labor, Bureau of Labor Statistics.

Gordus, Jeanne Prial, Paul Jarley, and Louis A. Ferman. 1981. *Plant Closings and Economic Dislocation.* Kalamazoo, MI: W.E. Upjohn Institute for Employment Research.

Hamermesh, Daniel S. 1987. "The Costs of Worker Displacement," *Quarterly Journal of Economics* 52,1: 51-75.

_____. 1989. "What Do We Know About Worker Displacement in the U.S.?" *Industrial Relations* 28 (Winter): 51-59.

Handbook of Labor Statistics. 1985. Bulletin 2217, U.S. Department of Labor, June.

Heckman, James, and Joseph V. Hotz. 1989. "Choosing Among Alternative Nonexperimental Methods for Estimating the Impact of Social Programs: The Case of Manpower Training," *Journal of the American Statistical Association*

Heckman, James, and Richard Robb. 1985. "Alternative Methods for Evaluating the Impact of Interventions." In *Longitudinal Analysis of the Labor Market Data*, J.J. Heckman and B. Singer, eds. Cambridge: Cambridge University Press.

Hirsch, Barry, and John Addison. 1986. *The Economic Analysis of Unions: New Approaches and Evidence.* Boston: Allen and Unwin.

Holen, Arlene, Christopher Jehn, and Robert Trost. 1981. "Earnings Losses of Workers Displaced by Plant Closings." CRC 423, Public Research Institute, Center for Naval Analysis.

Jacobson, Louis. 1977. "Earnings Loss and Job Loss Due to Employment Reductions in the Steel Industry." Ph.D. dissertation, Northwestern University.

_____. 1978. "Earnings Losses of Workers Displaced from Manufacturing Industries." In *The Impact of International Trade and Investment on Employment*, William G. Dewald, ed. Washington, DC: U.S. Department of Labor, 87-98.

_____. 1984. "A Tale of Employment Decline in Two Cities: How Bad Was the Worst of Times?" *Industrial and Labor Relations Review* 37: 557-69.

_____. 1988. "Structural Change in the Pennsylvania Economy." Report, W.E. Upjohn Institute for Employment Research, Kalamazoo, MI.

_____. 1991. "The Dynamics of the Pittsburgh Labor Market." Report, W.E. Upjohn Institute for Employment Research, Kalamazoo, MI.

Jacobson, Louis, Robert LaLonde, and Daniel Sullivan. 1992. "Earnings Losses of Displaced Workers." Working Paper, W.E. Upjohn Institute for Employment Research, Kalamazoo, MI.

Johnson, Terry, et al. 1986. "An Evaluation of the Impact of ES Referrals on Applicant Earnings," *Journal of Human Resources* 20, 1 (Winter): 117-87.

Jovanovic, Boyan. 1979. "Job Matching and the Theory of Turnover," *Journal of Political Economy* 87, 5: 972-90.

Katz, Arnold. 1990. "Length of Joblessness and the Employment Service: Philadelphia and Pittsburgh Workers Receiving Unemployment Benefits 1979-87" Unpublished mimeo, Department of Economics, University of Pittsburgh, February.

Kletzer, Lori. 1989. "Returns to Seniority After a Permanent Job Loss," *American Economic Review* 79,3: 536-41.

176

_____. 1991. "Earnings After Job Displacement: Job Tenure, Industry, and Occupation." In *Job Displacement: Consequences and Implications for Policy*, John T. Addison, ed. Detroit: Wayne State University Press.

Kosters, Marvin. 1986. "Job Changes and Displaced Workers: An Examination of Employment Adjustment Experience." In *Essays in Contemporary Economics Problems: The Impact of the Reagan Program*, Phillip Cagan, ed. Washington, DC: American Enterprise Institute.

LaLonde, Robert. 1986. "Evaluating the Econometric Evaluations of Training Programs with Experimental Data," *American Economic Review* 76, 4: 604-620.

Lazear, Edward. 1981. "Agency, Earnings Profiles, Productivity, and Hours Restrictions," *American Economic Review* 71, 4: 606-20.

Leigh, Duane E. 1990. *Does Training Work For Displaced Workers?: A Survey of Existing Evidence*. Kalamazoo, MI: W.E. Upjohn Institute for Employment Research.

Lerman, Robert I. 1982. "A Comparison of Employer and Worker Wage Subsidies." In *Jobs for Disadvantaged Workers: The Economics of Employment Subsidies*, Robert Haveman and John L. Palmer, eds. Washington, DC: The Brookings Institution.

Lewis, H. Gregg. 1986. *Union Relative Wage Effects: A Survey*. Chicago: University of Chicago Press.

Madden, Janice F. 1988. "The Distribution of Economic Losses among Displaced Workers: Measurement Methods Matter," *Journal of Human Resources* 23, 1: 93-107.

McLaughlin, K. 1991. "A Theory of Quits and Layoffs With Efficient Turnover," *Journal of Political Economy* 99, 1 (February): 1-20.

Meyer, Bruce D. 1992. "Policy Lessons from the U.S. Unemployment Insurance Experiments." NBER Working Paper 4197.

Mincer, Jacob, and Boyan Jovanovic. 1981. "Labor Mobility and Wages." In *Studies in Labor Markets*, Sherwin Rosen, ed. Chicago: University of Chicago Press.

Murphy, Kevin M., and Robert H. Topel. 1987. "The Evolution of Unemployment in the United States: 1968-1985." In *NBER Macroeconomic Annual 1987*, Stanley Fisher, ed. Cambridge, MA: MIT Press.

Neumann, George. 1978a. "The Direct Labor-Market Effects of the Trade Adjustment Assistance Program." In *The Impact of International Trade and Investment on Employment*, William Dewald, ed. Washington, DC: U.S. Department of Labor, No. 87-98.

_____. 1978b. "The Labor Market Adjustments of Trade Displaced Workers: The Evidence From the Trade Adjustment Assistance Program." In *Research in Labor Economics*, Vol. 2, Ronald G. Ehrenberg, ed. Greenwich, CT: JAI: 353-81,

Owen, Bruce, and Ronald Braeutigam. 1978. *The Regulation Game*. Cambridge MA: Ballinger.

Podgursky, Michael and Paul Swaim. 1987. "Job Displacement and Earnings Loss: Evidence From the Displaced Worker Survey," *Industrial and Labor Relations Review* 41: 17-29.

President's Advisory Committee on Labor Management Policy. 1962. *Benefits and Problems Incident to Automation and Other Technical Advances*. Washington, DC: Government Printing Office.

Ruhm, Christopher. 1991a. "Are Workers Permanently Scarred by Job Displacements?" *American Economic Review* 81, 1: 319-323.

_____. 1991b. "The Time Profile of Displacement-Induced Changes in Unemployment and Earnings." In *Job Displacement: Consequences and Implications for Policy*, John T. Addison, ed. Detroit, MI: Wayne State University Press.

Seitchik, Adam, and Jeffrey Zornitsky. 1989. *From One Job to the Next: Worker Adjustment in a Changing Labor Market*. Kalamazoo, MI: W.E. Upjohn Institute For Employment Research.

Shapiro, Carl, and Joseph Stiglitz. 1984. "Unemployment as a Worker Discipline Device," *American Economic Review* 74: 433-44.

Stiglitz, Joseph. 1974. "Alternative Theories of Wage Determination and Unemployment in LDCs: The Labor Turnover Model," *Quarterly Journal of Economics* 88: 194-227.

Swaim, Paul, and Michael Podgursky. 1991. "The Distribution of Economic Losses Among Displaced Workers: A Replication," *Journal of Human Resources* 26, 4: 742-755.

Tannery, Frederick J. 1991. "Labor Market Adjustments to Structural Change: Comparisons Between Allegheny County and the Rest of Pennsylvania 1979-87." Unpublished Working Paper, Economic Policy Institute, University of Pittsburgh.

Topel, Robert. 1990. "Specific Capital and Unemployment: Measuring the Costs and Consequences of Worker Displacement." Carnegie-Rochester Series on Public Policy, No. 33: 181-214.

_____. 1991. "Specific Capital, Mobility, and Wages: Wages Rise with Job Seniority," *Journal of Political Economy* 99,1: 145-176.

Woodbury, Stephen A., and Robert G. Spiegelman. 1987. "Bonuses to Workers and Employers to Reduce Unemployment: Randomized Trials in Illinois," *American Economic Review* 77, 4 (September): 513-30.

U.S. Bureau of the Census. 1988. *Current Population Survey, January 1986: Displaced Workers*. Ann Arbor, MI: Inter-university Consortium for Political and Social Research.

U.S. Office of Management and Budget. 1991. *Budget of the United States Government*, fiscal year 1991.

Index

184

Swaim, Paul, 23, 25

TAA. *See* Trade Adjustment Assistance
    (TAA)
Temporary layoffs, 7, 92-94
Tenure
    pre- and postseparation earnings loss
        with, 100
    as predictor of earnings loss, 28-29
    returns to, 26-30
    See also High-tenure workers
Topel, Robert H., 2, 24, 27, 30, 31-32,
    33, 152
Trade Adjustment Assistance (TAA)
    as income replacement program, 140-
        41, 144, 151-52
    under Trade Act (1974), 2, 3, 12-14
    under Trade Expansion Act (1962),
        13
Trade competition impact, 2, 12-18
Training and retraining programs
    Area Redevelopment Act (1959), 2
    costs of, 156
    duplication of, 158
    under EDWAA, 155
    effectiveness, 170
    evaluation, 155-56
    under Pell Grant, 157
Training services programs, 140-41
Transportation workers, 121
Trost, Robert, 16, 17t

UI. *See* Unemployment insurance (UI)
Unemployment insurance (UI)
    to assist displaced workers, 140-41,
        144

collection rates by workers
    approaching separation, 92, 94, 98
current system, 161, 169
earnings losses of noncollectors, 94
income replacement, 149
proposed alternatives, 161
See also Emergency Unemployment
    Benefit (EUB) program;
    Employment Service (ES);
    Extended Benefit (EB) program;
    Reemployment bonus
U. S. Department of Defense,
    Community Adjustment Program,
    159
U. S. Department of Labor
    Bureau of International Labor Affairs
        (ILAB) studies, 11-19
    Bureau of Labor Statistics, 19
U. S. Office of Management and Budget
    (OMB), 3

Wage subsidy program, 160-69
    See also Earnings subsidies
Women
    earnings comparison with men, 98-99
    pre- and postdisplacement earnings
        loss, 92, 98, 118-20t, 124
    predisplacement tenure effect on
        earnings, 28-30
Woodbury, Stephen, 163
Worker dislocation. *See* Displaced
    workers; Earnings losses
Worker earnings alternative models, 51-
    56

Zornitsky, Jeffrey, 23, 51

About the Institute

The W.E. Upjohn Institute for Employment Research is a nonprofit research organization devoted to finding and promoting solutions to employment-related problems at the national, state, and local level. It is an activity of the W.E. Upjohn Unemployment Trustee Corporation, which was established in 1932 to administer a fund set aside by the late Dr. W.E. Upjohn, founder of The Upjohn Company, to seek ways to counteract the loss of employment income during economic downturns.

The Institute is funded largely by income from the W.E. Upjohn Unemployment Trust, supplemented by outside grants, contracts, and sales of publications. Activities of the Institute are comprised of the following elements: (1) a research program conducted by a resident staff of professional social scientists; (2) a competitive grant program, which expands and complements the internal research program by providing financial support to researchers outside the Institute; (3) a publications program, which provides the major vehicle for the dissemination of research by staff and grantees, as well as other selected work in the field; and (4) an Employment Management Services division, which manages most of the publicly funded employment and training programs in the local area.

The broad objectives of the Institute's research, grant, and publication programs are to: (1) promote scholarship and experimentation on issues of public and private employment and unemployment policy; and (2) make knowledge and scholarship relevant and useful to policymakers in their pursuit of solutions to employment and unemployment problems.

Current areas of concentration for these programs include: causes, consequences, and measures to alleviate unemployment; social insurance and income maintenance programs; compensation; workforce quality; work arrangements; family labor issues; labor-management relations; and regional economic development and local labor markets.